Surfing the Waves of Alzheimer's

Principles of Caregiving That Kept Me Upright

RENÉE BROWN HARMON, MD

MANY
HATS
PUBLISHING

Published by Many Hats Publishing, Birmingham, Alabama
www.reneeharmon.com

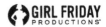

Edited and designed by Girl Friday Productions
www.girlfridayproductions.com

Design: Paul Barrett
Project management: Sara Spees Addicott

Image credits: cover photograph courtesy of the author,
cover wave pattern by Shutterstock/natsa

Lyrics from "Surely the Presence of the Lord" copyright © 1977
Lanny Wolfe Music (ASCAP) (adm. at CapitolCMGPublishing.com)
All rights reserved. Used by permission.

Portions of the first two chapters were previously published
as a personal essay, "Learning to Surf," reproduced with
permission from *JAMA Neurology*, 2019; 76(1):11-12.
Copyright © 2019 American Medical Association. All rights reserved.

ISBN (paperback): 978-1-7347917-0-9
ISBN (ebook): 978-1-7347917-1-6
Library of Congress Control Number: 2020905483

First edition

"You can't stop the waves, but you can learn to surf."
—*Jon Kabat-Zinn*

To Harvey: my rock, my touchstone, my heart.

Introduction

The Heart Never Forgets

When my husband, at age fifty, was diagnosed with Alzheimer's disease, our world was irrevocably changed. Our previously charmed life, each piece of it fitting in its place and perfectly balanced, became swamped, and we were left scrambling for footing. Our family was thrust into an ocean of churning waves. How was I going to stay afloat and upright?

I have always admired the grace and beauty of surfers gliding along mountainous waves and through beautiful cerulean tubes—specks of humanity juxtaposed against the majesty and awesomeness of nature. And they made it look so easy. My long-ago eight-year-old self was enamored with *ABC's Wide World of Sports* and its variety of human athletic achievements. Surfing was one of my favorites to watch: the sun, the waves, the tan bodies sailing effortlessly along a wave. I was entranced and wondered if I would ever get the chance to try it myself. I finally got that chance on a family vacation to Costa Rica in 2009.

It was our first full day there, and we were scheduled to have surfing lessons. Let me tell you, it is not as easy as those professional surfers make it appear. For our first lesson, our instructor had us lie belly-down on our boards with our hands holding the board at shoulder level. Then we were to go from that position to a low squat in one motion. The teenagers and children in our family had no difficulty, but most of us over a certain age just could not do it! The instructor then took said teenagers out into the surf for the next step—performing that maneuver in the water. Not wanting to be left onshore with the grown-ups, I decided to take my board into the water and watch the proceedings from a better vantage point. The water was not too rough, I reasoned. I was wrong. A wave washed over me, my feet were swept off the ocean floor, and I went under. My board, which was attached to my ankle via its leash, smashed into my left shoulder. I managed to get back to the shore and the grown-ups (more grown-up than me evidently!) without anyone noticing my graceless attempt to just walk into the ocean with a surfboard. But the crushing ache in my shoulder was excruciating, and I had to lie down on my board, nauseated and sweating with pain.

I am a family physician, and I knew that I could diagnose myself with a careful examination. As I lay on my board, I did just that. I could move my shoulder, but it hurt when I put it through all ranges of motion—no shoulder dislocation. My collarbone was not tender to palpate and felt normal—no clavicular fracture. I could flex at the elbow and shoulder, and there was no tenderness at the insertion of the long head of the biceps—no tendonitis or tendon rupture. Now, how about the AC joint? Yikes! There it was. I had dislocated my acromioclavicular joint! The most common scenario for this kind of injury is a bicyclist who wrecks, is catapulted over the handlebars, and lands directly on the top of the shoulder. Evidently, my surfboard had hit me squarely on that point. It wasn't a horrible injury; I wasn't going to need to go to a Costa Rican emergency room. All I needed was ice and ibuprofen, but it was going to prevent me from enjoying some of the activities we had planned for the rest of the trip. More importantly, it was the harbinger for what later turned out to be the more terrifying moments of our vacation—when I realized that something was wrong with my husband's cognition.

This book will take you, the reader, through my journey of finding a diagnosis for my husband, how the disease affected him, our family, and our friends, and on to his journey's end. It was eight long years, but the years were filled with joy and richness, as well as obvious struggle. I've organized the book roughly chronologically, but also thematically. I found it impossible to tell our story in a purely chronological manner; I would have had to update the reader on my husband's abilities and losses at each stage of the disease. Instead, I have chosen to take a theme, such as driving, and describe the evolution of said theme over time.

Early in the process of contemplating this book, I was asked to speak at our local Alzheimer's Foundation yearly gathering and educational event, Alzheimer's in Alabama. I was honored to be asked to be the lead speaker of the daylong event, with instructions to speak for forty-five minutes on my "thoughts about Alzheimer's." That's all the guidance I was given! How in the world was I going to speak about dementia for forty-five minutes? As I began preparations for my talk, I organized my "thoughts" around principles of caregiving that I had learned and picked up along the journey. I realized that I could tell some personal stories to illustrate some of these principles, and then explore them in further discussion. I ended up with a dozen or so such principles. I arranged them in a somewhat linear manner and ended up with material that greatly overshot the forty-five-minute time allotment. My presentation was well received, but I felt as if I had only scratched the surface of the material that was our story. I had been journaling during the entirety of my husband's disease; I had a wealth of stories and maybe a modicum of insight to share. This book was born!

Each chapter is titled using one of the principles I have discovered. Some lessons were stated outright or asked of me in exactly the form presented here. One of the first that I read and held on to as a maxim came to me as I was searching the internet for information about Alzheimer's disease: "If you've seen one case of Alzheimer's disease, you've seen one case of Alzheimer's disease." I was looking for a clear delineation of what to expect going forward, but the answer I got was, essentially, "Your experience will be yours and yours alone." It wasn't very comforting at first, but as I met more people on this same path, I realized that each of our stories was different, and there is a certain beauty of humanity in that sentiment. Other principles came from my support group. I especially responded to "It's better to be kind than correct" in dealing with a person with dementia. Our group emphasized this point multiple times through the years, with each other and with first-time visitors. Friends have unwittingly contributed other chapter titles, as have my husband's physician and my counselor. As I examine these principles now, I am struck by how universal many of them are to all of us as human beings. Of course it is better to be kind than correct! Imagine how seamless our interactions could be if each of us managed to lean into that statement! Every special education teacher would tell you that his or her students "aren't giving me a hard time; they are having a hard time." And yes, it's important to keep your loved one with dementia active, but we should all stay active.

See what I mean?

Now, a word about my choice of words. My husband was diagnosed officially with "younger-onset dementia, probably of the Alzheimer's type, early stage." My patients often ask me what the difference is between dementia and Alzheimer's disease. I've had several people say some variation of, "My father has dementia, not Alzheimer's." Dementia is an umbrella term that denotes difficulty and abnormalities in cognition but says nothing about the root cause of the problem; it's a symptom, not a diagnosis. I like to illustrate this difference by saying, "Fever is a symptom of an illness, but the term 'fever' doesn't say what its cause is. Dementia is similar. It means there are cognitive issues, but it doesn't say anything about their cause." Alzheimer's disease is the most common cause of dementia, accounting for about 50–70 percent of all cases of dementia. Vascular dementia, caused by multiple small strokes, is the second most common, at about 20 percent. Other less common causes of irreversible dementia are Lewy body dementia, frontotemporal dementia, Huntington's disease, and Creutzfeldt-Jakob disease. *Mixed dementia* is the term used to name cases that have aspects of two or more causes. With good neurologic testing and follow-up, most cases of dementia can be categorized, but a definitive diagnosis can only be conferred at autopsy. It is not the scope of this book to explore the science behind the diagnosis of Alzheimer's, nor of its treatment or future therapies. I leave it to the reader to explore these topics on their own or with the guidance of their personal physician. Because of the confusion many have with the terms *dementia* and *Alzheimer's*, and because many readers of this book may have a family member with a diagnosis of dementia of a different cause, I do use the words interchangeably. It is my hope that this does not cause further confusion, as it will necessarily conflate the terms. Rather, it is my attempt to include all causes of dementia, thus speaking to all readers.

I also struggled with what term was most appropriate for talking about persons with dementia or Alzheimer's disease. When I first wrote "you should include your person with dementia in daily life" or "keep your person active," it sounded too impersonal. I have, therefore, elected to use either "your family member" or "your loved one." I realize that some readers may be professional caregivers, but I would hope that they view their clients as "loved ones." And it is my hope that readers without personal knowledge of dementia will be able to identify with most, if not all, of my expressed ideas and sentiments, and just experience the story.

So why this book? How is this book different from other books about dementia and Alzheimer's disease? First, Alzheimer's disease is a looming public health crisis as our baby boomer population ages. At present, approximately 5.8 million Americans are living with Alzheimer's disease, about 10 percent of the population aged sixty-five and older, with that percentage expected to rise to 14 percent by the year 2025. It is likely that every person in the US knows of at least one person with Alzheimer's disease. And thankfully, there is an abundance of good literature and information available to patients and family members affected by this disease. Books like *The 36-Hour Day* have been "must reads" for caregivers for years. There are also a great number of well-received books, movies, memoirs, blogs, and podcasts dealing with the daily travails of dementia.

Second, what I have attempted to do here is combine the genres of a "how-to" and "memoir" into a category termed *teaching memoir*. It is my hope that my personal accounts, followed by a brief discussion of the topic addressed in each chapter, will lead the reader to a deeper reflection of their own journey with Alzheimer's disease. Then, using the concluding practices, the reader can reach even deeper. It is also my hope that as a physician, I am able to offer a clear-eyed account of our story, and in fact, I may sound too clinical and removed at times in my telling. Believe me, I have felt "all the feels" that each of you caregivers have felt. The reader may also rightly wonder if an account of someone with younger-onset Alzheimer's disease can be applicable to all ages and causes of dementia. I assure you that younger-onset Alzheimer's disease manifests itself just like its older-onset counterpart. Granted, it is much rarer; only 3–5 percent of all Alzheimer's disease patients are diagnosed before the age of sixty-five. A younger patient experiences some unique difficulties, which I will illustrate, but there are universal truths to be gleaned from anyone's account of living with this disease.

One of those universal truths is that anyone can learn to surf in an uncertain world! I may have gotten rocked by the waves and thrown into the ocean of dementia, but I eventually did learn to ride those waves and keep my balance. I didn't do it all by myself; I had friends and family who taught me how to stay upright and supported me when I seemed about to capsize. I learned to trust my instincts in caring for my husband, just riding the waves, but I also relied on the wisdom of other caregivers' words and writings. If I felt that I was sinking, swamped by my emotions and the never-ending list of things that needed to be done, I would metaphorically drag myself out of the ocean and lie down on my surfboard for a bit— taking a walk, playing the piano, reading a poem. It is my hope that by reading these stories and essays, you, too, can take that first step onto a surfboard and learn to ride the waves of whatever ocean you find yourself in.

My Perfectly Balanced Life

I think that I may have the world's largest corpus callosum. Let me explain. The corpus callosum is the structure in the brain that connects the two halves of one's brain, transporting information between the two hemispheres. And how do I know, you might ask, that mine is so highly developed? Well, most people will tell you that they are either predominantly right brained or left brained. That's really lovely—to be able to fit the idea of one's brain and identity in that nice neat box. I'm simplifying terribly, and neuroscientists everywhere are quaking when I say this, but one's right brain is more occupied with creativity, the large picture—it's artsy-fartsy; the left brain is logical and detail oriented. To help remember the distinction between the two, think of a capital letter *R* with its curvy top and the letter *L*, all straight lines and right angles. One is either predominantly right brained or left brained. Not me. I could never categorize myself that way. And it was maddening growing up not being able to classify myself as either logical or artistic. I like it all! I want to understand it all! I am even good at most things I try, never excelling at any one thing in particular. I love math and puzzle games, and I love creating art—visual, musical, written.

I come by this balance of my two brain halves naturally. My mother is a retired teacher of elementary students who are gifted, and my father is a retired mechanical engineer. They are perfect examples of pure right- and left-brain predominance respectively. My two younger sisters are each an embodiment of one of the hemispheres: one is an accountant, the other a singer and real estate agent. In school, I was on the mathematics team as well as the literary magazine staff. Even my hobbies are a blend of both. Playing the piano requires precise movements and skill in translating the little black marks on a sheet of music into something your fingers do—like typing, actually. But without the right brain to create nuances in dynamics and tone, maybe even bringing an emotional feeling to a piece, playing music could be a purely mechanical exercise. Quilting combines geometry and a feel for color to create beautiful works of art. The first two college courses that I selected to take during the summer between my junior and senior years in high school were Human Growth and Development and Art History. Even my chosen career, family physician, is a highly complex mix of scientific facts and intuition, the art of medicine. Yes, I could conceivably plug your symptoms into a computer and come up with a diagnosis, but because I know what you do for a living, your family makeup, what medications you take, how much alcohol you drink, and more importantly, how you carry yourself, your coloring, the tone of your voice (and on and on), I can develop a more nuanced differential diagnosis and have a better idea about what treatment options might work best for you.

It's been helpful to realize this fact about myself. It explains why I find so many different subjects fascinating and why I like to wear so many hats. I fully embrace the fact that I am a dilettante! So how have I kept all these spinning plates from crashing? I created a perfectly balanced life for myself, one where I had the time and space to be spouse, mother, physician, friend, student, reader, musician, and artist at the same time. I couldn't have managed to pull that off without Harvey, my husband since 1985, cheering me on, supporting me, and giving me that time and space to cultivate all my diverse interests.

Harvey. He was one of those rare people who knew, at the age of ten, exactly what he wanted to be when he grew up: a physician; and he pursued that goal relentlessly and methodically. He was from a working-class family; his mother worked at the Social Security Administration, his father as an entrepreneur with a string of ventures he was always chasing. And because his father, Bill, was frequently traveling, his mother, Lois, managed the household. Harvey's brother, Dennis, was four years older, and they weren't particularly close growing up as they were quite different in temperament. Dennis was loud and argumentative, skirmishing with his mother about her rules, and chafing under her supervision. Dennis also loved debate and excelled on the debate team, even coaching high school teams while in college. I think Harvey learned from watching the battles between his mother and brother to be quiet and obedient and fly under the radar. When they were children, their physical habits were different as well. Dennis would spend his time reading, while Harvey rode his bicycle, shot hoops, and roamed the neighborhood with the family collie, Rusty. As different as the brothers were, this nuclear family believed in the power of a good education. Both Dennis and Harvey attended a magnet county high school for students with high IQs. Dennis became a lawyer, and Harvey, influenced by his family's own beloved doctor, became the quintessential family physician, pursuing that dream with dogged determination.

My own family of origin was also squarely middle-class, living in a suburb located geographically beside the one Harvey lived in, though we never met, as we were zoned for different school systems. My school system was a little more affluent. I struggled to fit in, as most adolescents do, but academic achievement wasn't particularly lauded by my classmates, so I was viewed as a bit of a nerd—math team and literary magazine, remember! Sometime in high school, I began to understand that I wanted a career that could blend my love of science with helping people, and I ran through ideas of physical therapy, dentistry, and medicine. I settled on dentistry when I applied to college, mainly because it appeared that all the other scholarship applicants were stating medicine as a career choice. I wanted to stand out, so I said that I would pursue dentistry. I got as far as actually applying to dental school before I realized that teeth and the mouth were too limited of a discipline for my expansive interests, and I switched to premed.

I met Harvey in college. Actually, I can't say that I ever *met* Harvey. When you go to a small liberal arts college, you just know everyone, especially if you're in the same sciencey premed classes. He was a year ahead of me, but during one semester, we had three classes together, including French. I remember that he asked me to join him in a study session once, but I turned him down because I didn't *need* a study session. He later told me that he had admired me from afar for a while and especially liked my "springy ankles."

"My what?"

"I like the way you bounce when you walk!"

He didn't ask me out again until after he had graduated and I was a senior—this time not to a study session, but to a Crosby, Stills & Nash concert. What I most remember about that first date was that he grabbed my hand and held on tight as we made our way through the throngs of people leaving the concert. He said that he didn't want to lose me in the crowd. We dated off and on after that, and I began to realize how kind and brilliant he was. And he had great-looking legs. But it wasn't until he returned home from a six-week trip to Europe, called me, and we talked for hours on the phone that I realized that I *really* liked this guy. He was so kind. And gentle. And patient.

We dated in earnest and fell in love. When we were both accepted into the same medical school in the same year, that clinched it for us as a couple, and we were married the summer after our first year of med school. I'm not sure I could have made it through medical school without Harvey's gentle, quiet spirit keeping my stress in check. He had such a calming influence on everyone around him, always did! In the third year of medical school, rotations in all the medical specialties were designed to help the students decide on a career choice. Harvey and I both chose family medicine, independent of each other, and for different reasons—I for the breadth of knowledge required (did I mention I have a lot of interests?), he for the better outpatient medicine training. We completed our residencies in beautiful Charleston, South Carolina, both of us selected as co–chief residents, then moved back to Birmingham, Alabama, our hometown, to practice medicine. These first seven years of marriage, medical school, and residency set the stage for our future life together. We were never competitive with each other, somehow managing to make the same grade point average, class rank, and even board certification scores. We instinctively knew we were two halves of a whole, equals, and set out from the start to make our lives together reflect that mutual respect and equality. We divided household chores—cooking, cleaning, and bill paying—neither of us playing into the myth of gender roles.

It probably comes as no surprise that we wanted to practice together. It was our goal to share the responsibilities of a family medicine practice as well as share the responsibilities of raising a family and managing a household. We would be co-owners, co-workers, and co-parents. When we started the

practice, Double Oak Family Medicine, in 1992, I was preg-
nant with our first daughter. The practice was brand-new, and
we were only seeing two to three patients a day, so it made
sense that one of us would be at the office, and the other would
be home with the baby. We alternated days at home and days
at the practice, so that we were each part-time physicians. We
eventually had two daughters, and they had the equivalent of a
full-time parent. As our daughters grew, our practice did too,
so that by the time they were in elementary school, the practice
could support both of us being at the office until one of us left
to pick up the car pool, then stay with the girls the rest of the
day. Our daughters had the advantage of being fully parented
by both of us. Our patients accepted this arrangement, most
choosing one or the other of us as their primary physician,
but agreeing to see the other if the schedule dictated it. Some
patients never had a preference and would easily float between
the two of us, as the charts held all the information both of us
needed. The staff had no problem working with both of us, as
we were so similar in our approaches. The ultimate plan for the
practice was for both of us to be full-time at the office when
our youngest daughter turned sixteen and could drive herself.

Logistically, the plan worked so that the one at home was
responsible for planning and preparing the family dinner,
ideally to be ready to eat when the one at the office called in.
Whoever was at the office would call home when they were
on their way, making it possible for the hot meal to be ready
when we walked in the door. Or, if we were running late at the
office, we would call the other as a courtesy so that the meal
wouldn't get cold. The noncook of the evening was responsible
for cleaning up after dinner. Breakfasts were Harvey's responsibility; lunches were mine. Whoever was home was responsible for helping the girls with homework and driving them to
their after-school activities. We each took responsibility for
getting one daughter ready for bed, then would read together

as a family—one Bible story and one fun story. Yes, we alternated the reading responsibility too, so that one of us wasn't seen as the "fun book" parent. Harvey did the majority of the yard work, and I did all the grocery shopping. The responsibilities at the office were shared as well; Harvey took on most of the financial planning, and I took on the personnel planning.

My time out of the office was spent being a mother at first, playing our small games, going to the library for books; but once the girls were in preschool, I relished my time alone by reading, going out for coffee with friends, shopping, and working on whatever creative project I was currently immersed in. I remember Harvey coming home and asking what I had done with my time off and feeling guilty after running through my litany of small pleasures. I'm not sure why I felt so guilty about it—maybe because I wasn't cleaning or cooking or being productive like a *good* wife would, societal norms still having a pull on me.

Harvey had a little harder time knowing what to do with himself when he was outside of the office; he much preferred to be practicing medicine. He was a wonderful father, though. Reading aloud to the girls, playing basketball with them, or coaching their soccer teams, he was a constant presence in their lives. I treasure memories of him playing horse, one daughter on his back yelling for "Baldy," Harvey's horse name, to gallop faster. Unfortunately, we don't have much video of Harvey, as he was the one usually behind the camera, even documenting the Cesarean section of our firstborn, and the vaginal birth of our second. He enjoyed working in the yard, planting a small vegetable garden each year. And there was the line of family dogs: Miss Kyle, Blackie, and Nash. Each dog knew to pick Harvey as his or her special person. They were *his* dogs. Running long distances eventually became his prime activity once the girls were in school.

Harvey was the consummate physician, even looking the part; tall and slender, with rimless glasses, button-down shirt, and tie, he always wore a long white lab coat, black stethoscope around his neck, pockets bulging with prescription pad and books. His patients loved him. He was kind, attentive, and patient, and the best listener I have ever known. Stories abound about his kindness and thoughtfulness. He once called a three-year-old on the phone after he had removed a particularly painful splinter from her hand, just to make sure she wasn't mad at him. Another patient told me that he once emptied his brown paper lunch bag so that he could place some sample medications in it for her. I know of at least three patients who credit Harvey with saving their lives—and never tire of telling me so. It was as if he was born to be a physician.

I'm not sure that I quite have his all-encompassing natural gift as a physician, but I still love what I do! I count it a vast privilege to be allowed into people's lives in such an intimate way, connecting in personal ways that only close family and friends are usually allowed. I love the detective work involved in solving mysterious symptoms. I love educating patients on a particular disease process and what they can do to alter its course. I especially love seeing my efforts have an impact on a patient's health, as they lose weight, get fit, have lower blood sugar readings, and just feel better. What I call the bread and butter of a family practice, sinusitis and bronchitis, is also rewarding when I stop to realize that by helping with these simple problems, I am relieving discomfort and making it possible for someone to return to work more quickly.

Our daughters were seventeen and fourteen years old when Harvey was diagnosed with Alzheimer's disease and have now grown into remarkable young women. Elena, the oldest, is a licensed clinical social worker who works for a housing program for young mothers experiencing homelessness. Elena is married to Brett, who works as a project manager for a company that pairs patients with health coaches. They met in college, and Brett moved to Birmingham, after graduating, to be with Elena. They have been married for two years and live two blocks down the street from me.

Christina is three years younger than her sister and is now a fourth-grade special education teacher in a local elementary school. Christina has been dating Phil since high school, and they seem destined to marry. Phil has just graduated from college and hopes to work in marketing. Christina, too, lives two blocks from me. Though Harvey and I were frequently asked if the girls were following in our footsteps as physicians, we knew it probably wouldn't happen. They are their own persons, and both daughters have proven to have big, big hearts for the most vulnerable among us. They make me so proud.

Like most people, Harvey and I had dreams and plans for the future. We could talk endlessly about what kind of neighborhood and house we would move to once the girls graduated from high school and we could downsize and not worry about school systems. Planning to retire at about age sixty-five, we wanted to travel and tossed around all kinds of ideas, usually involving adventure and activity. Our family vacations had mostly featured national parks, and we dreamed of extending that type of travel to other countries, exploring the diversity of other cultures and landscapes. We considered that our daughters, once they graduated from college, would probably choose not to live in Birmingham. We would travel to visit them and their possible new families in whatever location they landed.

All of our lives have been changed by Alzheimer's disease, Harvey's more than anyone else's, of course. The rest of this book details the changes we all experienced: in him, in ourselves, and with each other. My perfectly balanced life was permanently thrown off-kilter with his diagnosis. I was going to have to rely on both halves of my brain to survive what was coming: left and right. My corpus callosum would need to kick into overdrive and achieve a new balance in a totally new life that would be constantly shifting. I would need to learn how to keep my balance while riding the waves that were sure to come.

❧

PRACTICE

1. Briefly describe your life before Alzheimer's disease. It was your life. It deserves to be told, so write it out or share it with a friend.
2. Create a music playlist of popular songs or hymns that you and your loved one enjoyed in the past. As you play the songs, let them transport you to experiences you shared.
3. List favorite aspects of your family that you treasured most before dementia arrived. Circle those aspects that still remain.

If You've Seen One Case of Alzheimer's, You've Seen One Case of Alzheimer's

My hands trembled, my heart raced, and I broke out in a sweat as I dialed the number. Who turns in their own husband as an impaired physician? Our state's medical licensing board has a phone number anyone can call anonymously to report a physician that they think may not be safe to practice medicine. I had been poking around on the board's website for over a month, looking to see what measures were in place for our particular situation. There was the anonymous tip line, and programs were available to help physicians who were struggling with addiction, but there was nothing on the website about my husband's particular plight. I called the board and said that I needed to talk to someone anonymously about my physician husband, who was also my partner in the medical practice we shared.

⟨⟩

It was during the big family vacation to Costa Rica in December 2009 that I had the first jolt of fear that something was wrong. Harvey had a hard time following our guide's instructions, asking me to remind him what we were to do. We went zip-lining high above the forest canopy, but he forgot to empty his pockets of his wallet, keys, and prescription sunglasses as we had been instructed. One night our seventeen-year-old daughter ran ahead of us to our cabin. I asked Harvey to go after her to help her find her way back. She was fine, but Harvey became lost and was found wandering the property forty-five minutes later by the resort staff. He had to be driven back in a golf cart in the pitch black. The last day there, I got up the nerve to tell him that I was concerned about him and asked him a few questions.

"In what year was Christina born?"

"Um, I don't remember."

"Well, she is fourteen years old, so what year would that make it?"

"I can't do that, Renée."

"Well, it was 1995, and if she was born in 1995, and Elena is three years older, in what year was *she* born?"

"Um, 1998?"

Wow! My brilliant husband, who was a fully invested parent, didn't know our daughters' birth years and couldn't perform simple math! I told him that I was very concerned about him and that I wanted him to see a neurologist when we got home. He wasn't keen on that idea, but struck a bargain with me. He would work on some brain-training games for two months, and if his scores did not improve, he would see a neurologist then.

In the following months after our Costa Rica vacation, I spent lots of time researching frantically on the internet for anything I could find about dementia. Because I knew. I just knew in my gut that this is what Harvey's problem was. He was forty-nine years old, though, and that piece of the puzzle wasn't adding up. Could he really have that rare condition, younger-onset Alzheimer's disease? I knew of it, but had never seen it in our practice. So I read. And the more I read, the more I was convinced that this is what was going on. I never told him what my explicit concerns were, and he never brought it up. He said that his scores had not improved in the two months he worked on his brain-training games, but forgot our bargain, and I had to cajole him into going to the neurologist.

The neurologist took our concerns very seriously, did a complete evaluation, and concluded that Harvey had mild cognitive impairment (MCI) based on the history she obtained and his slightly poor score on a memory screening tool. He also showed some mild atrophy on a brain MRI, and slowing of his brain waves on an EEG. She placed him on Aricept immediately. I remember being confused that she was starting a medication without a diagnosis of dementia, and I hadn't ever heard of MCI. So, back to the computer I went, armed with this new term.

MCI is a descriptive term, exactly as it sounds. Clinically, it implies that only the patient and/or a person close to the patient notices a problem. It doesn't impact the patient's life. MCI can stay as MCI, or it can progress to dementia—meaning that the cognitive problems begin to impact daily life and become noticeable to others.

Of major concern to me as soon as I realized that Harvey was having memory issues was whether and when he should stop practicing medicine. The term *MCI*, and its definition, which included the word *mild*, reassured me, but how would I know if his memory issues impacted his practice? Yes, we shared a practice, and I was with him in the office every day, but I wasn't in his exam rooms with him. I couldn't secretly tape his encounters. Harvey himself reassured me that he was fine to practice. But would he really be able to judge that? The neurologist was less than helpful with her response when I asked, saying only, "You'll just have to keep a close eye on him." After Harvey had the diagnosis of MCI, I became hyper-alert to any signs he might exhibit at work. He began to ask me simple questions when we were at the office together, seeking my opinion a little more than he usually did. One particularly shocking question floored me.

"Now, how do we treat poison ivy?"

As the months progressed, the questions increased, so I asked him if he felt like he could still practice. He said that he had no difficulty with easy cases and just referred patients to specialists when he didn't know what was going on. When I pointed out that even simple problems sometimes gave him difficulty, he confided that he sometimes relied on his medical assistant to help him.

"How does she help you, Harv?"

"She helps me remember what medications to use."

Like the poison ivy question! But it was advice from a nonphysician. If I happened to see a patient that Harvey had previously seen, I would read his note to see what had trans-pired. His notes were getting sketchier and shorter, just basic information.

And staff didn't report anything to me! I thought surely the medical assistant that worked most closely with Harvey, helping him remember medications, would say something to me, but she never did! Actually, there were a few general con-cerns from the staff. "Is Dr. Harvey OK?" or "Dr. Harvey seems a little lost today." I evaded these comments and never asked staff directly if they noticed any changes in him. I guess I was trying to protect him, shield him, not betray him, and there was probably a measure of denial on my part. How long could I put this off? Mostly, I was a stew of anxiety.

And when I'm in a stew, I tend to research. This is when I first stumbled on the state medical licensing board's website, almost frantic for help, but not wanting to divulge our secret. So one afternoon when I was home alone, the kids at soccer practice, Harvey at the office, I dialed the anonymous tip line. Through strangled breath I spelled out the problem: my medical partner had been diagnosed with MCI and I needed help in figuring out how to know if/when he shouldn't practice. The partner thought he was fine to continue. And by the way, the partner is my husband.

It turned out that I was speaking to a lawyer at the board (yikes!), but he was incredibly kind, understanding the untenable position I was in. He said we needed a clear answer to this question; maybe another specialist could write a note to the board stating Harvey had MCI, but it wasn't affecting his ability to practice medicine. We decided that I needed an outside source to make that determination, that it was unfair to ask me as his spouse to do that. I relayed that the neurologist had been shy of helpful in this regard, and I wasn't sure how to get this determination. The phone call ended with me feeling validated, and with a goal of trying to figure out the next step.

Ensuing research led me to the discipline of neuropsychology. I knew of the field, if only obliquely. As I delved further, I found that the large teaching hospital in Birmingham, the University of Alabama at Birmingham (UAB), had a very good department and that it had ties with the Memory Disorders Clinic there. I read about the types of testing they did, the types of disease processes they studied, and their staff. I discovered that the head of the department had a special interest in MCI and even younger-onset Alzheimer's disease. I emailed this neuropsychologist, outlining our situation and asking if this type of testing could help determine Harvey's ability to practice medicine. He didn't respond until two weeks later because he was out of town, an agonizing two weeks for me.

During these two weeks of waiting, I had a distressing encounter with an angry patient. She was an X-ray technician in a local hospital, relatively new to the practice, with no chronic medical problems, who was in to see me about a bronchial infection. When I walked into the room, I found her pacing the small space, almost bursting with indignation. She spluttered that she was thoroughly disgusted by the care she had received the week earlier from Harvey. She would normally have seen me, but evidently chose to see Harvey then because I was out of the office. I listened as she ranted that Harvey didn't seem to know what he was doing. It was that vague. The only concrete complaint she had was that he asked her what antibiotic she preferred and then forgot what she had told him a few minutes later. On the pure face of it, there just wasn't much there. Had I not known that he had cognitive issues, I would have been very perplexed at the vehemence she exhibited. She even demanded a refund for that office visit. I'm sure it was because she didn't know Harvey well; his loyal patients would never have said something like that to me. In any event, that encounter shook me out of my lassitude and mobilized me to doggedly pursue the next step.

He had a follow-up appointment with the neurologist the next week, and I told her that a patient had complained to me about the care she had received from Harvey, but that it was minor and not apt to lead to a lawsuit. I told her that I thought neuropsychological testing would be helpful at this point, and that I would like her to pursue a referral. She suggested someone in private practice, but I pushed for the department at UAB. She agreed, and I soon got a response to the email that I had sent earlier to this neuropsychologist, instructing me how to set up an appointment.

All of this was done covertly behind Harvey's back, and I felt guilty as hell about it! But I was getting nowhere with him when I tried to discuss it. I'm sure he felt ambushed at this point, but I tried to couch it as concern for his patients, and he did agree that he never wanted his cognitive disability to cause harm to a patient. He had no recall of the angry patient when I asked him about that encounter, and he continued to state that he could see the easy patients and refer the difficult ones. I couldn't get into his brain, so I can only imagine the turmoil he must have been feeling, knowing his memory was declining, but trying to hang on to his identity as a physician.

In preparation for the neuropsychological testing, we were mailed a ten-page questionnaire that both of us were to fill out. In response to the question "What do you want to learn from this testing?" Harvey wrote, "I want my memory back." I had to pester him to add "and can I still practice medicine?" We answered what seemed like unending questions about his prior health, medications, level of education—all very thorough. We mailed it in and waited to hear about the appointment.

The day of neuropsychological testing finally arrived; it was six weeks from my initial contact with them. As we drove to UAB, we listened as usual to National Public Radio. As we pulled into the parking garage, StoryCorps came on. An older couple told the story of the husband's Alzheimer's disease and his wife's loving caregiving. It was touching and sweet on its own, but I listened in dread. Harvey commented when it concluded, "That wasn't too bad."

Sitting together in the waiting room, we were the only people there. We were both interviewed separately, and I was able to lay out all of the issues and problems I was seeing and witnessing. It was very thorough. I don't know what Harvey's interview was like. The bulk of the day was spent with Harvey undertaking numerous tests of his memory—verbal, spatial, numeric, logical. It was exhaustive, and he was exhausted. He was able to tell me a little of what it entailed. He thought he probably failed, and was defeated. It broke my heart when he told me that it made him feel stupid.

It took a month for the neuropsychological testing to be scored and compiled, and we went back to UAB to hear the results. All of the tests were explained, as were his scores, with statistics on how he compared to normal subjects of his age and level of education. I was stunned by the breadth of testing that was done. No wonder he had been exhausted! The results of each of the tests were mounting into what I could tell was much more abnormal than I had anticipated. Harvey had been doing an exceptional job at hiding his disability. It was stunning how poorly he had performed.

After the results were explained, the neuropsychologist stated that Harvey had dementia, probably of the Alzheimer's type. Harvey broke down and sobbed. I didn't cry; I think I knew what was coming, and was not surprised, and probably just relieved to have a diagnosis! But it broke my heart to see him broken. After he recovered, the neuropsychologist then said that Harvey shouldn't practice medicine any longer. Harvey sobbed again, and when, in just a few seconds, he seemed to quiet down a bit, the neuropsychologist said, "It's OK, take all the time you need." Harvey immediately straightened his back, looked the guy straight in the eye, and with a steeliness I rarely saw said that he was fine to go on. We were then told that we should call the medical board, and they would tell us how to gradually transition Harvey out of the practice.

That was a late Friday afternoon, near the end of September 2010. We spent the weekend telling our family—our daughters, his parents, my parents, his brother—and just digesting the news. As I said, I was much further along in this process, but it seemed to be all new to Harvey. I remember trying to bring up subjects related to longer-term planning and how he angrily dismissed me: "Renée, I'm fine! I don't want to talk about it." We discussed ways he could spend his time now that he wasn't going to be working as much, and eventually not at all. We brainstormed, but really couldn't come up with much—he just didn't have any outside interests except for long-distance running. Maybe he could take up guitar?

Late Monday morning, after I had seen my last patient, I called the board, explaining the final diagnosis and position from the neuropsychologist—that Harvey shouldn't practice medicine. I said that I was told that the board would help me formulate a plan to transition Harvey out of the practice. It was actually the same lawyer that I had spoken to previously. He hemmed and hawed a bit, then got another lawyer on the line, and I said my part again. Pretty quickly, I was told that Harvey needed to leave immediately and not see another patient. Ever. I was really taken aback and asked again if there wasn't a way to ease him out.

"No, ma'am, he needs to stop immediately. It's too great of a liability for him to continue."

I asked if he could just see his afternoon patients that were already scheduled. No. Now. So I told Harvey, then we told our practice manager. It was lunchtime, so at 12:45, when the staff was coming back, we called a staff meeting, and Harvey, through tears, told the completely stunned and unsuspecting staff about his diagnosis. Then he went home. When I left that evening, I caught a glimpse of his long white lab coat, with his stethoscope in its pocket, hanging on the back of his office door, and sobbed.

Not only did we not have a transition plan that day, but our beautifully balanced life plan was destroyed. All in a moment, I was given—no, I was thrust into—a new life plan, one that had me as a full-time solo physician, the primary parent to two teens, with full responsibility for a household, and caregiver to my husband.

Let the surfing begin.

☙

I've just told you the story of how I knew that Harvey was having memory issues and how it impacted his career as a physician.

Our story is uniquely ours; no one has a story exactly like ours. Your story is uniquely yours. Each case of Alzheimer's disease is different because every person is different. When a disease affects the brain, and because our brains are uniquely ours, what results is unique to the individual. When you compare stories about your loved one with someone else who is caring for a dementia patient, this truth is obvious. Not all patients repeat questions endlessly; not all patients wander; not all patients become belligerent. You see what I mean. You are living with, or caring for, one person, one unique person, and you will need to approach care in a way that is uniquely geared to that one person.

There are still commonalities seen across the disease spectrum. It does pay to educate yourself about the stages of the progression of Alzheimer's, even if every patient doesn't necessarily follow a strict path of progression. You will have a better idea of what to expect in the coming years, and what typical behaviors might arise. I recommend reading as much as you can, from reputable sources, but as you read, beware of claims that Alzheimer's can be cured. There is no cure at the present.

I found it particularly helpful to watch YouTube videos. Seeing a real-life person in the different stages of the disease made what I was reading come to life. I remember watching an interview of a couple, the husband with dementia, and thinking, *This is how we will be in a few years; Harvey smiling and present, with me doing all the talking.* I wasn't far off. There are disturbing videos out there too, but they can help you learn what *not* to do. I watched a video of a man trying repeatedly, for more than fifteen minutes, to get into a car, with no one helping him! What was the point of recording that poor man's struggles?

cso

PRACTICE

1. Tell *your* story. At least a part of your story. Tell it to a trusted friend, or write it in your journal. You might choose to tell how *you* became aware of your loved one's memory problems. You might choose to tell how your life has altered from your previous life. You could tell about a particularly sweet interaction with your loved one. The story is yours and your family member's, but it needs to be shared.

2. Create a timeline of your journey with dementia, marking important dates and time periods, emphasizing the uniqueness of your particular journey.

3. If you are more visually oriented, try imagining this timeline as a journey on a map. Where are the mountains, valleys, rest stops, scenic overlooks, or long stretches? What is your compass?

If You've Seen One Case of Alzheimer's, You've Responded to One Case of Alzheimer's

Before our Costa Rica trip in 2009, about two to three years prior, Harvey kept bringing up, laughingly, that he thought his memory was getting bad. He wondered if he had been so laid-back during his life that he hadn't engaged his brain enough to keep it healthy. I didn't see it myself and thought it was just middle-age worry.

Then he started getting on my nerves. We had been equal partners all our married lives; now it seemed that I had a much greater role in managing the family calendar. I had always been better at it, knowing where everyone was supposed to be on a given day, but I thought he knew all this too. Was I oblivious to my own control over this factor of our lives for all the years the girls were younger? Was I so good at it that he abdicated the responsibility entirely to me? I would constantly review the plans for the day in my mind, making sure I could get everyone to where they needed to be. When a change occurred in the daily routine, I would intensify my efforts at running the schedule through my brain. Eventually, I became resentful and angry that he just didn't seem to care, wasn't engaged in our lives enough to care, and couldn't be bothered by the minutia of adolescent comings and goings. He would ask me questions about the girls' lives and schedules that we had already discussed and planned for. He was supposed to know all this; he had been told. It felt like he just couldn't be bothered to remember it! I quit telling him about upcoming family weekend plans, preferring to spring it on him, just so that I didn't have to hear the refrain, "You didn't tell me that."

About a year and a half prior to our Costa Rica trip, he needed to plan a solo trip to Massachusetts to run the Boston Marathon, and he asked for my help. I didn't want to help him; this was his trip, and he could plan it on his own! It took him a long time, but he did put all the pieces together for the trip, and managed to pull off making all his air and ground connections. I had only a vague concern that something might not go well, but was mostly relieved that he could actually do this without me.

Once Costa Rica happened and I knew that something was wrong with my husband, I immediately took to the internet to see if what I was witnessing fit with a diagnosis of dementia. The more I looked, the more I was convinced that this was the case. I would have moments of doubt, especially if he came up with a brilliant point in conversation or a patient praised his abilities, but mostly, I just *knew* this was what was happening to Harvey. The emotions I felt at this time were primarily grief and anger. As I tentatively looked into a future in which Harvey was afflicted with dementia, I felt tremendous loss for him personally. Who would he be if he weren't "Dr. Harvey"? Being a physician was his purpose. It's what he inhabited so easily and had longed for and pursued so relentlessly. What would he do without that? Somehow, I instinctively knew not to bring it up to him. We had only vague conversations at this time about his "memory problems" and how he might work to improve them. Maybe I knew that he wasn't ready to look ahead to possible futures. I don't know, because we never talked about it. So I stewed in my anxiety alone. Of course, I also experienced grief for myself and our daughters. Even in the early days, before a definitive diagnosis, when I *knew* we were looking at probable dementia, I found myself projecting into the future and becoming grief-stricken, thinking that our daughters may not have their father at college graduations or there to walk them down the aisle at their weddings. We wouldn't be traveling together as an older adult couple. We wouldn't even get to be empty nesters. I would likely have a giant baby bird in my nest instead.

And I was mad! Mad as hell that my perfectly balanced life was going to be upturned and that I would have to be responsible for everything. I would become the Queen of Everything, responsible for running the household, parenting, and all financial decisions. We had worked so hard to achieve that balance, and now my balancing partner, the other end of my seesaw, would be stepping off, leaving me to somehow manage it all. The hardest change I had to digest and come to terms with was that I would have to become the only physician at Double Oak Family Medicine—a solo physician at that! I loved, and still do love, being a physician, but I also deeply treasured my time off, pursuing all my various interests. How would I do it all? What was I going to have to give up just so that I could keep all the balls in the air? I knew I could do it. I am a strong woman, born that way and raised that way. But I didn't *want* to do it all! This is not what I had signed up for. And it was going to worsen as time progressed, with me doing more and more with each passing year. I was resentful as hell, and he hadn't even been diagnosed yet.

Interestingly, I was never angry at Harvey for getting this disease. That just never crossed my mind; it was completely illogical. I did have great anger at him for not talking about his diagnosis. He never did talk about it, not just at this very early stage in knowing something was going on, but ever. And that angered me immensely. Not only was I going to have to be in charge of everything, I couldn't even talk about it with the person I was closest to. I couldn't openly grieve in front of him. I was going through this horrific thing without "my person." Sure, it would not have been fair of me to burden Harvey with my grief and anxiety when he was probably suffering his own, and I suspect we were both extremely lonely in our individual grieving. But mostly, my response to Harvey through all this was always great sorrow for him.

I was never angry at God either. My faith is not built on the idea of a God who directs what happens to humanity, one person at a time. I have never believed in a God who chooses to afflict certain people with certain diseases or directs weather events to harm a certain population. God cares about us and loves us and grieves along with us. I believe that God set this world into motion at creation, and life just happens. People get sick, tornadoes occur, brakes fail, but God is not directing it all in some grand scheme, pointing a finger at this person or that and commanding cancer to enter a body, for example. There may be some grand plan that none but God understands, but I cannot believe that God is micromanaging creation on a day-to-day scale. I did, and still do, get angry at a theology that wants to say that God had a purpose in Harvey's disease, or that everything happens for a reason. A song we sing at church includes the line, "All things come together for my good." What possible good to Harvey is there in having dementia? I can digest the idea that our daughters and I may see some good out of this, but for Harvey? No.

Harvey and I wanted our daughters to be fully aware of what was going on. I had been talking with each girl as soon as I knew that their dad was having some memory problems. They had been noticing a few things too, and would say, "Sometimes Daddy just doesn't make any sense." "Those brain-training games don't seem to be helping him much." "You better come pick me up, Mom. I don't think Daddy could find it." All said with a wink and a chuckle. Their silly father. They weren't taking it very seriously. I wondered if they were just experiencing the usual adolescent awakening to the foibles of their parents. But I wanted them to know that we were taking this seriously, and that what they were noticing, we were noticing as well. When I told Christina that her grandmother would be picking her up at school because we had an appointment with a neurologist, she asked, "About Daddy's memory?" When I told Elena about the upcoming appointment, she asked more questions, even "It can't be Alzheimer's, can it? He's too young!" I pressed her a little further, and she admitted that she was somewhat worried.

We had a family meeting, right after Harvey's first neurology appointment, four months after our Costa Rica trip. Each of us sitting in our favorite spot in the den, I asked Harvey to start off by telling them what had transpired at the appointment. I wanted them to know that we wouldn't keep secrets from them, and that I didn't want to talk to them about it behind their father's back.

"The doctor told me that I do have some problems with my memory and did some tests. They took some blood, and I'll be doing some X-rays and brain scans, then we'll meet again with her to go over all the tests. I might not be able to be a physician at some time in the future, but that won't be a financial problem. Your mother will still work, and we have good disability insurance. We'll still be able to pay for your college educations and future weddings."

(Eye-rolling from the daughters.)

"This is not something you should talk to your friends about, or your grandparents; we need to keep it between the four of us."

Elena was shocked at this and asked, "Why won't you be telling your parents about this?"

"Because it would devastate them."

After the follow-up appointment with the neurologist to discuss all the testing that had come back showing some abnormalities in his brain, I told each girl that the tests were looking like it was a serious issue. Christina nodded and went about what she had been doing, because at fourteen, she really just didn't understand. Elena cried and asked, "What does that mean, Mom?"

"We can't be certain yet, but he has mild cognitive impairment, and it might turn into something worse."

"Like Alzheimer's? Will he not know us eventually?"

"Oh, sweetheart, it will be many years before that happens, if it ever does. We still don't know, and remember, he is taking medicine to slow this down."

"And he still isn't telling his parents about this?"

"No. That's up to your dad, but he thinks it would be too hard on them, especially since we don't know anything definitive yet. Please know that you can ask me anything, talk to me about what you're thinking and feeling. We can't go through this alone."

And she dissolved into tears as I hugged her. After the definitive diagnosis was made through neuropsychological testing in September of that same year, Elena responded with more worry and concerns about going away to college. Christina still didn't have much of a response; she didn't even know what Alzheimer's disease was. There was no way that she understood what the future held. She would be living with it for the next four years; she would learn.

When we finally got confirmation that Harvey did indeed have Alzheimer's disease, in the car on our ride home I asked him who he thought we needed to tell. Straight out, he said, "Our family." When I asked him who that meant, he said, "My parents, Dennis, the girls, your parents and sisters."

Because he had always said that he didn't want to tell his parents, I was surprised and asked, "What do you want to tell your parents?"

"That I have Alzheimer's."

I was confused at his change of mind, but I surmised that these were the people who loved him best; he wanted them to know.

The next day, we went to his parents' house, ostensibly to watch a football game, and told them that we had news to share. We were sitting at their kitchen table, eating the pizza that we had brought for dinner, and Harvey just flatly stated, "I have Alzheimer's disease."

His mother, Lois, was predictably devastated, and repeatedly said, "I don't see anything wrong with you, Harvey. Are you sure? You seem the exact same to me." Then she tried to come up with family members that might have passed on this disease to her son, saying that no one in her family had dementia, but pointed out that Bill's mother had had it. Lois was obviously relieved to be able to point the finger of blame at Bill's side of the family. This was typical of his parents' exchanges at the time—a bit contentious. After she had settled that in her mind, she asked Harvey, "Can you still drive?"

"Yes, of course. I can still do most things. I just can't work." But she wouldn't let it go and kept asking about the driving. Bill was quieter and sadder, obviously taking in the news with gravity. Harvey told them that they would be seeing a lot more of him in the future, as he planned to visit them frequently.

Harvey's brother, Dennis, was coming into town the next day, so we planned to visit at their parents' house again in order to tell him of the diagnosis and to ask his legal opinion about how Social Security disability worked. However, Lois told Dennis about Harvey's diagnosis before we got there, but I didn't know it, and as we sat awkwardly in their parents' den, waiting for Harvey to tell his brother that he had dementia, Dennis jumped right in and asked, "So, the two of you have some questions about Social Security disability?"

"Um, so you know that Harvey has Alzheimer's?" I asked.

"That's what I've been told."

Harvey just nodded as I fumbled with my basic questions about disability, my mind scrambling to figure out exactly what Dennis had been told. He seemed cold and skeptical as he launched into lawyer mode, explaining the details of applying for disability. Then he casually dropped a bombshell.

"I had a client once who had dementia. Turns out that he was being slowly poisoned with mercury by his wife. Has Harvey been tested for heavy metal poisoning?"

Realizing that Dennis's only source of information about Harvey's diagnosis was whatever his parents had heard from us, held on to, and told him, I launched into an explanation of the neuropsychological testing. With Harvey sitting there, shrinking in his seat as I talked about how poorly he had performed, I tried to establish the validity of the diagnosis and deflect the thinly veiled accusation that I was somehow behind this diagnosis and was trying to make a grab for my husband's disability checks! In the car, on the way home, I turned to Harvey as it hit me, and in amazement said, "I think Dennis just accused me of poisoning you!" Harvey just chuckled and said, "That's Dennis!"

We told my parents and sisters, and they were all very kind and sad and supportive, later privately offering me reassurance that they would help out as much as they could. Harvey didn't want our friends to know, but I had to share the diagnosis with my closest friends because I realized that I needed their support and care, especially if Harvey continued to refuse to talk to me about any of it. Actually, while away for a trip with my three closest girlfriends just before his first neurology appointment, I did tell them of my mounting concerns. It was a vast relief to spill out my worries. I find it very difficult to bottle my anxieties, and by sharing, I was also looking for confirmation that my concerns were warranted. I told them what had happened in Costa Rica and what I had observed since then and asked, "Does that sound worrisome to you? Am I blowing this out of proportion?"

This closest group of girlfriends was a lifesaver for me. I didn't tell any of our friends from church until a year or so had passed, and even then I told them privately and asked that they not let Harvey know that they knew. No one ever treated him or our family any differently, even after his dementia was clearly apparent. I quietly let some of our other friends know, and with the exception of only one longtime friend, no one deserted him.

After Harvey was officially diagnosed with Alzheimer's disease and told he could no longer work, my practice manager at the office and I scrambled to find the most appropriate way to let our patients know. We worried that it would open us up to possible lawsuits if we announced his diagnosis; a disgruntled patient might see his diagnosis as an opportunity to place blame for a poor outcome. We chose instead to say that he had retired "for medical reasons." We sent a letter to all the patients that he had seen in the last eighteen months and fielded phone calls for weeks and months as they called to ask what had happened. Most of his patients chose to stay with me and the practice, but a few, mostly men, chose to find another physician. I am not exaggerating when I say that every day after his retirement, at least one patient asked me how he was doing, some even saying, "I miss Dr. Harvey." When they said that, I knew what they meant, but some worried that the statement would sound as if I weren't their physician of choice and would hurry to add, "But I like you too, Dr. Renée." I reassured them that I missed having him at the office too. At the one-year mark of his retirement, I decided that we could talk about his actual diagnosis if it came up. I had been asked to speak at a women's retreat for an area church, and I used this opportunity to share some of our story and make it official. All of our patients felt great sorrow for Harvey and his diagnosis. "He's so young!" "How did you know?" "How is he doing?" "Does he still know you?" All the usual questions people ask when a diagnosis like this is known. And it opened the floodgates for personal stories of their own about parents, siblings, and friends with Alzheimer's disease. It was mentally and emotionally exhausting to have these conversations every day, multiple times a day, but it also served as a wonderful reminder that these patients and this practice were indebted to Harvey and that I had really big shoes to fill.

∾

I titled this chapter similarly to the previous one because I wanted to show that not only is each person who is afflicted with Alzheimer's different from all others, but the people around that person will respond differently as well. Some will be shocked, some sad, some angry, some scared. As a caregiver to your loved one, you will likely experience all of those emotions at various times throughout the course of the disease. Own them. They are your emotions. They are valid emotions for the situation. You are not a bad person if you feel anger at your family member for having this disease, even if you know it's not a rational thought. It's even OK to be angry at God. God is big enough for your anger.

You will have to learn how to deal with the emotions of others too. I frequently comforted friends and family who were grieving over Harvey's diagnosis. That was a bit surreal. I found it frustrating at other times that when someone asked me how Harvey was doing, it was really a vehicle for them to tell me about their loved one with dementia. I would sigh inwardly, nod, and listen to their concerns. Often, as with so many other difficult situations, people just don't know what to say. Some may even avoid you and your loved one, thinking it too difficult emotionally. I really didn't experience this, but I have certainly heard many stories about friends and even family members that respond to this diagnosis by checking out. You will have to learn to accept that if it happens; you can't force anyone to respond in the way that you would prefer.

℘

PRACTICE

1. Name your emotions. Write them down in your journal. Explore them. What are you really angry about? What scares you? What makes you most sad?
2. How have those around you reacted when you shared the diagnosis? How did their reactions make you feel? If you've had anyone exit from your life because of this diagnosis, write a letter to that person (then throw it away!) telling him or her how you feel.

He's Not Giving You a Hard Time, He's Having a Hard Time

About a year and a half into his diagnosis, Harvey's mother, Lois, was diagnosed with Alzheimer's disease by the same neurologist and neuropsychologist who diagnosed him. His father, Bill, had already been diagnosed with an unknown type of mild dementia. They were both slowly declining and needing more help than they were willing to ask for. To his credit, Harvey's brother, Dennis, stepped up and took responsibility for his and Harvey's parents, traveling from Mississippi most weekends. It was not without confrontation, as he eventually had to take over their finances and make decisions on their behalf as their power of attorney. By this time, it was very apparent that Harvey could not oversee his parents' affairs, and he was never asked to, thankfully, and neither was I. However, the relationship between Harvey and his parents continued to be fulfilling for the three of them. Harvey would frequently visit them, giving them all some much-needed social interaction.

Two months after Lois's Alzheimer's diagnosis was official, she began falling. I received a call toward the end of my office hours one day from Lois's sister-in-law. "How is Lois doing?" she asked.

"Fine, as far as I know."

"Well, I heard she was in the emergency room and just wanted to check on her."

"She's in the ER?"

"Yes, she fell and hit her head. Bill and Harvey took her in."

Great! The elderly deaf man with mild dementia and the middle-aged man with dementia took the elderly falling woman with dementia to the ER without telling anyone! When I arrived at the emergency room, Lois was getting the last staple in her bleeding scalp. And then we all went home.

She fell two days later when her legs gave out on her, and she slid down the wall. Dennis was visiting, and when she still could not walk the next day, he took her to the hospital, where she was admitted for a full evaluation. The workup was unrevealing, so she was transferred to an area rehabilitation hospital four days later for a two-week stay to see if intensive physical therapy would help her safely walk again. Harvey and Bill visited her each afternoon, and Bill now had a sitter, Josephina, with him every morning. Josephina managed his medications, cooked his meals, and did light housekeeping. Harvey told me that the daily afternoon visits between Lois and Bill were sweet—Bill holding Lois's hand, telling her that she would be coming home soon if she worked hard.

Three days into Lois's rehabilitation hospital stay, I got a text from Dennis:

They are transferring me to UAB. I have a 4 cm mass on the left side of my brain, near the skull.

What the heck is wrong with this family's brains? I immediately called him back, but his secretary answered because she was the one who had actually sent me the text. She told me that Dennis had been unable to communicate effectively all day. Incorrect words kept popping up; he repeated the same nonsense over and over as he tried to express what he wanted to say. A friend had convinced him to go to the emergency room, and scans there found the mass. He was transferred from the hospital in Mississippi to our large teaching hospital in Birmingham, the University of Alabama at Birmingham, UAB, the same hospital where Harvey and Lois's neurologist was based. It was a glioblastoma and needed to be excised. He and his wife have a friend in Chicago who recommended a neurosurgeon there, at Rush University Medical Center, so all of his scans were sent there in preparation for surgery.

While Dennis was back home in Mississippi, preparing for surgery in Chicago, still having language difficulties, I got a frantic text from Dennis's wife, Jane.

Rehab hospital is releasing Lois tomorrow! Social worker says that Bill and Harvey told her that everything was arranged for her to go home.

Why do people try to communicate important messages by text? I called Jane and got a more detailed explanation about what had happened. The case worker had gotten the order from the physician that Lois was to be discharged the next day, and asked Bill and "the son that was with him" if arrangements had been made for her care at home. They answered, "Yes!"

Jane asked, "Are you saying that the son who has dementia just gave you his OK?"

"He has dementia?" asked the social worker. "He said he was a doctor and assured me everything was in place for Mrs. Harmon's discharge."

"Did you read the chart first? That son has dementia. And so does Mr. Harmon. You have to talk to the other son, Dennis. He's the only one who handles their affairs."

So Jane and Dennis, from their Mississippi home, arranged for Lois to be transferred to a nursing home in a bedroom community about an hour away from Birmingham. Lois's sister, who was also in declining health, was living there, and Dennis thought that even though she would be farther from Bill, it would be nice for Lois to be with her sister. She would be safely ensconced there, being taken care of by professionals while Dennis had brain surgery in Chicago, recovered, and then would be able to make long-term plans for both of his parents. Bill had Josephina to provide care for him, and Harvey would continue to visit him each afternoon. I was in charge of Bill's medications, setting up his pill container each week.

Dennis's surgery went well. He was kept awake during surgery, talking to a speech pathologist while the four-centimeter malignant glioblastoma was excised. They kept up a running dialogue so that the neurosurgeon would know if significant language difficulties arose, and surgery would then cease. Dennis retained most of his verbal skills after surgery, and continued to improve while he recovered in Chicago. He had gaps in his vocabulary, though, making conversation interesting as he would circle around the word he wanted until he or the person he was talking with was able to retrieve it. "Squirrel" became "the small woodland animal with nuts" and "bed" became "the place you lie down with pillows." He still has some of the same language issues today, but has been able to continue his law practice. Texting is how he and I usually communicate, and it can be entertaining and amusing, sometimes confusing and frustrating.

With everyone stable in Chicago, the nursing home, and Birmingham, I made plans for a quick beach trip over the Labor Day weekend. Josephina was also taking a mini vacation that weekend, so I planned for Harvey to visit with his father each of the days that we were gone. I got a text from Dennis my first day at the beach.

Dad tried get mom out of place she is in

What happened?

Dad drove to mom place with old people to get her out

By himself? Did he succeed?

Alone. The people not let him. Friend got him

So Bill drove to the nursing home to try to bring Lois home, but the staff wouldn't let him do it? What do you mean that a friend got him?

They put him in room. Friend drove to him and got him back

I don't understand.

Friend Ron went to the place drove Dad home

OK, your friend Ron drove to the nursing home, got Bill, and drove him home? Is that right? What do you mean by "put him in a room"?

Yes nursing home people put Dad in room and locked

They locked him in a room until your friend came to get him? What happens to Bill's car now?

Yes I dont care

To this day, I'm still not completely clear about what happened. What kind of room did the nursing home staff lock Bill into? Is that even legal? At least there was no mention in these texts that Harvey was involved in the shenanigans, so I called home to check on him and see what he knew. Maybe he could further flesh out this story. He knew nothing of his father's attempt to spring his mother from the nursing home or how Bill got home. I was no closer to understanding what actually happened, but at least Harvey wasn't involved. Until the next day.

Harv and dad tried again

Oh, no! What happened?

They drove to get his car and get mom

Harvey drove your dad to the nursing home so that Bill could get his car? Is that right? How did they try to get your mom out again? Surely they didn't let them!

Harvey said he was doctor and no they not let them

Yikes! Harvey pulled the doctor card again. I guess the nursing home knows about Harvey's diagnosis? Did they get home ok?

Dad drove his car and Harv followed

I called home after getting this text story to hear Harvey's version of it. He said that Bill needed his help to get the car, and they tried to bring his mom home, but "they wouldn't let her out until Monday." I had actually called Harvey throughout the day to check in and make sure he wasn't being pulled into the saga, so I was blindsided by the story Dennis tried to tell me. Evidently the nursing home administrator called him both days to report the goings-on.

I drove home from the beach the following day, Sunday, calling Harvey periodically, but he never answered. I assumed he had gone to church, but he still wasn't answering my calls in the midafternoon. He wasn't at home when I got there, but there was a pitiful-sounding message on the answering machine from Lois: "Harvey? It's your mother. Please call your father so you can both come get me." I called Bill's house. Harvey answered and told me that he and his dad had gone to visit Lois after church and the nursing home still wouldn't release her. Deciding I needed to at least try to better understand what had been happening all weekend, I drove to Bill's house. Bill corroborated what Dennis had told me about the last two days, then turned to Harvey and asked, "They said we could get her out tomorrow, didn't they?"

Harvey nodded. "I think that's right."

I began to explain why this wasn't a good idea. "Lois can't walk and is in a wheelchair and will need help getting in and out of the chair to the bed and to the toilet. Who is going to take care of her if you bring her home?"

"I guess I will."

"Bill, you're just not strong enough to lift her. We don't have anyone lined up to care for her. It would be much better for her to stay in the nursing home where they can help her."

"But! . . . We've been married for sixty-two years. I'm her husband. We're supposed to be together. I can't just leave her there without me. Dennis thinks I can't do anything. Harvey is the only one that understands! He is so helpful and pleasant to be around. Not like Dennis."

Harvey alternated between looking confused and nodding in agreement with his father. And I sat there thinking, *Yeah, Harvey does whatever you ask of him because he can't think for himself; he just wants to please you. He can't refuse you when you ask for help. Of course you think he's "pleasant"!* That evening, I got a long text from Dennis.

> **I am done. Dad and Harvey are going to get mom out and bring home. Nothing I can do to stop. Wash my hands of it all. I have to rest after surgery. Too much. They will do it anyway. I tried. If bad happens, not on me. Josephina will quit and dad see he can't do by self. Sorry. Call adult protective services private if bad happens.**

> Dennis, I am so sorry! I don't know what to say except I can't let that happen! I am responsible for Harvey, and I don't want him taken advantage of this way by your dad. But I have to work. I can't monitor him. He just wants to help; he doesn't understand.

> **Good luck. Done**

> Guess I'll see what tomorrow brings. *sigh*

This was a disaster waiting to happen. Bill, Lois, and Harvey were each safe in their respective, current situation, but I couldn't keep them from trying to alter it. Lois would continue to plead with Bill to bring her home. Bill felt like they should be together. Harvey just wanted to help. It would be completely unsafe to bring her home. Josephina would quit, they didn't own a wheelchair, and Bill had trouble remembering to take his medications, much less remembering to give Lois hers. They would call Harvey to help out, but what help could he realistically give? Someone was going to fall and break something or someone would take too little or too much of a medication. And now this whole mess was on me! I understood that Dennis couldn't manage the situation while recovering from brain surgery in Chicago, but I still felt abandoned. There was no one else to call on.

The next day was Labor Day, Josephina was back on duty, and everything fell back to normal. Except, when she arrived, Bill told her that he had brought Lois home. Josephina knew otherwise, but still had to search the house to convince Bill that Lois was not there. She called me, and I called the nursing home to confirm that Lois was still there. Then Bill told Josephina that he had fallen the night before and was in pain. She took him to the emergency room, where he was found to be dehydrated and to have a broken rib. Harvey and I did not visit Bill that day, Harvey saying that he didn't want to get involved, but I knew that as soon as either of his parents asked anything of him, he would not and could not refuse. He couldn't see that they were unintentionally manipulating him and using his dementia to their advantage. To be honest, they probably couldn't see it either. And Harvey couldn't see their situation clearly enough to make appropriate decisions for them.

A week later, Lois's sister died at the nursing home, and Harvey decided he needed to visit his mother again. I was at work and called to check on him when he told me of his plans. I begged him not to go, but if he did, to please carry his cell phone. He forgot both requests and drove the hour's distance. Josephina and Bill were already visiting, so I texted Josephina to ask her to look out for Harvey; maybe he could follow them home. However, Harvey had not arrived by the time Josephina and Bill left the nursing home. He made it there and back without any problem evidently, but he wasn't home when I got home from work. He strolled in at 6:30, perplexed to find me almost completely unraveled with anxiety.

Just two days later (this is now two months since Lois first went into the hospital and Dennis was diagnosed with a brain tumor), Harvey was scheduled to be seen for an examination prior to enrolling in a drug study at UAB. I was going to see patients in the morning, then take him in for this evaluation. My hopes were riding high that we might see some response from this study drug, but the first step was to make sure he qualified for the study. I got a frantic phone call from Josephina in the morning, while I was seeing patients at the office, saying that Harvey and Bill were planning to drive to the nursing home to try yet again to spring Lois. It was hard to understand all she was saying because of the high drama in her voice, but she was clearly upset.

"I can't take care of him and her both! You can try to pay me $900, but I can't do it."

I reassured her that the nursing home knew not to release Lois into Bill's care and that if they did, I was prepared to call adult protective services. She put Harvey on the line, and I reminded him of the important appointment later that afternoon and asked him again to be home and ready to leave after I left the office. He assured me that he understood the plan and would be ready. I asked, shakily, "Are you and your dad planning to visit your mom today? Because you really don't have time."

He replied with regret and sadness, "No, she can't come home now. Dennis says there are no plans in place yet to take care of her here. He says maybe in one month."

I wrapped up my morning, then drove home to pick up Harvey and drive to UAB. Only Harvey was not there! I called Josephina to see if she knew when Harvey had left Bill's house. Maybe he was on his way home and this important appointment could be salvaged. Josephina replied to my query, "I *told* you they was going to the nursing home to bring Miss Lois home. They done left out the back door in Mr. Harvey's car. That's how they did it!"

"But," I answered, "I just talked to Harvey a little while ago and he understood they couldn't do that! And he has a really important appointment. He was coming straight home!"

"Well, they done gone now!"

After I calmed down a bit, I called the nursing home, and was reassured that Harvey and Bill were there, and that, of course, Lois was not going to be released. They put Harvey on the line, and he had no recollection of our previous conversation and no knowledge of the appointment at UAB. When he returned home, he said contritely, "I'm sorry I screwed up your day."

One month later, now three months since Dennis's surgery and Lois's hospitalization, care was in place for both of Harvey's parents in their home, and Dennis was home in Mississippi. Of course, Lois didn't come home without some drama. Bill was getting agitated that it was taking a long time for the nursing home to discharge her on the appointed day, so he decided to drive there and speed up the process. Josephina detained him, which angered him greatly, so much so that he fired her. Dennis refused to intervene, so I was drawn into the drama again to smooth things over among the warring parties. Josephina said that she would come back if Bill agreed, so I negotiated the peace agreement. This delayed Lois's discharge date, but two days later, she came home. They now had around-the-clock care in the home, Dennis was back to practicing law, and I could concentrate my energies on keeping Harvey safe and happy.

ల

When Harvey and his dad set off to liberate Lois from the nursing home, they weren't out to make my life or Dennis's more complicated than it already was. Bill just wanted Lois home. Harvey just wanted to please his parents. Throughout this story, Harvey would agree with whoever was talking to him, be it me, Bill, or Dennis. In the moment, he seemed to understand and react to what was presented to him in the most logical and pleasing way he knew how. That was at Harvey's core—to do what was asked of him, kindly. But he would forget what he had been presented with and would move on to the next request as if it were the first. He couldn't process all the points of view that were given him sequentially. And it was extremely frustrating for me, thinking that he understood that it was impossible to bring Lois home and then finding an hour later he was in the car driving to the nursing home. It felt like he was deliberately trying to drive me crazy!

Yes, dealing with someone with Alzheimer's or other forms of dementia can be very challenging. It can sometimes feel like they are trying to sabotage your life. "Why are you doing this to me?" Caring for someone with dementia takes a lot of mental and emotional energy, so that when your family member does something that requires you to "fix" it, the focus beam of your frustration lands easily on him or her. They are making our lives so much harder just by virtue of being who they are now! And we know that's not fair. It's not their fault. It's the disease. But in the moment, the one causing our distress gets the brunt of our ire.

How much better it would be to step away for a moment and consider what this inciting incident was like for our loved one. Her brain cannot process her surroundings like yours can, and she is doing the best she can with the limited mental resources she has. She may find herself in a situation that she cannot completely understand, so she takes her cues from those around her.

She's not giving you a hard time, she's having a hard time. Try reorienting yourself to her point of view. What does this situation look like and feel like for her? In my story, Harvey's point of view was just wanting to please whoever was asking something of him.

જ

PRACTICE

1. Remember a difficult moment of caregiving, when your loved one seemed to be making your life particularly burdensome. Write a brief summary of what happened as you lived it. Now rewrite that story from your loved one's point of view. Write it in first person, even. My rewrite might go like this:

   Renée has left me alone for the weekend. When my dad calls to ask me to pick up his car at the nursing home, I gladly agree. It's the least I can do. He's my father. When we get to the nursing home, Mom begs to come home and Dad asks me to talk to the staff. I tell them that I am a doctor and that we are ready to take her home. The nursing home staff says we can't. So we go back home. Renée calls me and she is angry. I don't know why she says we can't bring Mom home and that I shouldn't have let Dad try. I don't know what she is talking about. Dad is angry that Mom is not at home. I am confused.

2. Consider carrying a small object in your pocket or placing it in a common area that will serve to

remind you to empathize with your loved one.
Examples might be a shell, a stone, or a coin.

3. Sit in your loved one's favorite chair, close your
    eyes, and imagine a twenty-four-hour period from
    his perspective.

It's Better to Be Kind
Than Correct

Harvey and I divided all our chores evenly, including bill paying. Since we each had a paycheck, we each had our own checking accounts, and we divided the bills so that we had an equal distribution of that as well. Did I mention that we were rather anal about our division of labor? Once Harvey's diagnosis was made, I knew that eventually I would have to take over paying all the bills and management of our accounts. Since I didn't know how he paid his bills— for example, which were automatic deduction, which he paid online, which he paid with a check—I decided that we should start paying all our bills together. I didn't tell him the reason I wanted to do this was because one day he wouldn't be able to; I just said, "Harvey, it's crazy that I don't understand all the financial things you take care of. Let's sit down and pay the bills together. Then you can show me where all our assets are as well, and how you access those accounts." (I knew how to access my IRA accounts, but he had his own, complete with passwords.) And that worked! We sat side by side at the large oak desk in our home office, and Harvey paid all his bills, I paid mine, then he showed me where to find his IRAs. I wrote down all the usernames and passwords for each account. The ensuing months, we followed the same routine. As the disease progressed, it became increasingly difficult for Harvey to even log on to the computer, so eventually I asked if I could pay his bills, but said I still needed his help. We sat down together at the desk, and saying, for example, "Now, for your credit card bill"—yes, we had separate credit cards!—"I remember we log on like this," I would continue through the steps, talking my way through it, asking for Harvey's assent that I was doing it correctly, even though I knew what I was doing at this point. Eventually, he lost all interest and ability to do any of it, but by then, I was proficient and confident that I knew how to manage all our household and retirement accounts.

Because I was at the medical practice every day, it fell to Harvey to get the mail at home each day. Using the system we had long established, he would open the mail, throw away the junk, and lay the bills and statements on the oak desk, stacking them in order of when each was due. It became my practice to come home from work and make a tour through the house, looking for items in wrong locations, checking table surfaces for papers, and checking the office desk for new mail and bills. I eventually began to find paperwork—bills and statements— scattered around the house, and would round them up and set everything in order. It became a game of sorts, playing detective. What am I going to find today? I began to find old statements lying on the desk—old credit card and bank statements from several years back, with items circled or crossed out. Later, I would find whole files emptied on the desk, their contents drastically rearranged, so that I would have to sort through and refile them all. It certainly was frustrating, but I never let on to Harvey. I devised ways to keep him out of the four-drawer file cabinet where all the statements were stored, going so far as to purchase a chain that I threaded through the handles and secured with a lock. He could still get into it! We had misplaced the key to the file cabinet, and I was on the verge of buying a whole new cabinet just so I could lock it. When I went to the office supply store to purchase one, the salesman there told me that I could purchase a key from the manufacturer, which I did, and voilà, problem solved.

But because I knew Harvey was finding some satisfaction in going through the files, circling and underlining, I began to call it his "paperwork," and left out old statements for him, asking him if he could work on some of it for me while I was at the medical practice. He would sigh and say that he would, and when I returned, I would find his handiwork scattered around the house and praise him for all his hard work. When Harvey began attending respite care, there were invariably activities that he didn't want to participate in—namely, arts and crafts! The staff quickly learned to give him some "paperwork," and he would contentedly toil away, circling and underlining.

One day, while I was seeing patients, I got an alert from the tracking device I had placed in Harvey's car by this point. I tracked him to the bank, then checked our online banking site, and saw that he had withdrawn $5,900 from his banking account, the exact amount of money he received monthly from his disability insurance. I called the bank, but was told that Harvey had already left, and that he had indeed withdrawn that sum. I tracked him back to the house and called Christina. Luckily, she was at home and agreed to intercept her father and see what he could tell her about his adventure at the bank. She told me that when he walked into the house, he held his hand out, holding a roll of cash, and said uncertainly, "I have this!" to which she replied, "That's a lot of money, Dad! Let's find a safe place to put it." They stashed it in the top drawer of his bedroom dresser, and he went to check on it periodically until he forgot about it. I had my drive home from work to think about how I would address the cash in the drawer without belittling him, so after dinner, I casually asked him if he had been to the bank.

"No! Why would I go to the bank?"

"Well, I was looking at our bank account and saw that someone took out $5,900, and I was wondering if you did?"

"Renée, I did not go to the bank!"

"Well, I'm wondering if you did and just forgot, so let's look around and see if we can find it. It'll be a treasure hunt!"

So I pretended to search the house, knowing exactly where the cash was hidden, with Harvey tagging behind me. Eventually we "found" it, along with the withdrawal slip.

It was not my best caregiving moment when I exclaimed, "Look, here it is! I was right! You DID withdraw this money from the bank!"

Harvey was chagrined; he had no recollection of going to the bank, withdrawing the money, or stashing it away. I explained that his disability check was automatically deposited, and we would need to get it back into the checking account. I don't think he understood.

The next day, Harvey and I went to the bank to deposit the wad of cash back into the account. At the teller's window, I explained that we needed to make a deposit. The teller recognized Harvey and discreetly asked me to follow her to a closed office space. Telling Harvey I would be right back, I met with the teller, who told me the story of what happened the day before. She said that he had approached her desk, laid the disability statement on the counter and said, "I need this." She intuited that he wanted to withdraw that amount, and because it was his account, gave him the money. With some hesitation, I told this total stranger that my husband had Alzheimer's disease and that I needed to speak to a manager to see if there was something we could do to prevent this from happening again. The solution was extremely troublesome and would have involved lots of hoop jumping, so I declined. I was able to do all this without letting Harvey know we were discussing him. Other financial situations arose over time. About a year into the disease, Harvey started asking me to check his calculations of the tip at restaurants, then over time, asked me to completely calculate it. Eventually, I just took the bill and paid it. He could pay for purchases with a credit card, until eventually he couldn't. He went through a spell about two years into the disease when he would decide he needed a particular expensive electronic item. He bought a nice digital camera, two iPods, and a video camera—none of which he could operate! It frustrated me greatly to come home and find these unnecessary purchases, and I would usually fly off the handle at him. I just can't stand wasting money! But a wise friend pointed out that it was just money and if Harvey seemed to get some joy from buying them, even if he didn't use them, what was the harm? Besides the large bank withdrawal, the scariest moment regarding money was when I came home and found a note he had scribbled from a phone call with the words, "Children's Wish."

"What's Children's Wish, Harvey?" I asked.

"They called and I said that I would help them."

"Oh! What is it that they do, and how are you helping?"

"I don't remember what they do, but they are going to send some information and an envelope for me to send money."

It wasn't the Make-A-Wish Foundation; it was an organization I had not heard of, so I googled it and found reports that more than 80 percent of their proceeds went to administration. Other people had registered concerns about them, and it really did seem shady. Luckily, when the envelope from this organization arrived, I found it, and saw that he was correct in saying that he had promised them money. He was to put the money in the accompanying envelope and send it back. I told

Harvey that I researched this group and that they didn't seem reputable.

"But I told them I would give them money," he replied. Instead of arguing, I discreetly threw it away, and when he asked about it later, I lied, and told him that I hadn't seen it. He soon forgot about it. I called this organization and asked to be taken off their call list, then went online to put our number on the National Do Not Call Registry.

 app

It was really hard for me to learn not to correct Harvey's wrong words and ideas. I often found myself standing to the side while Harvey was in conversation with someone, and if he said something preposterous, I would shake my head vigorously so that the other person would understand that what he was saying was not correct. Of course the other person knew that! But it's really difficult to stand there and listen to someone say something completely off the wall or even just a little wrong. It was easier when it was just the two of us; I guess because there was no reason to be embarrassed. My daughters have chided me for always wanting to be correct, and I admit that I have been known to correct the grammar of strangers (rarely), and will argue a point when I know I'm right. Once he was diagnosed with dementia, Harvey's mode of interacting with friends and relatives was to nod and agree with most anything; that's when I would stand to the side and shake my head.

A person with Alzheimer's disease just cannot understand reality as we see it; they are trying to make sense of a world that often doesn't make sense to them because they cannot lay down new memories, and they are relying on their older memories. When they say odd things or ask questions, it isn't necessarily our job as caregivers to explain the truth. Often they can't handle the truth. And really, what would be gained by trying to get them to understand the truth?

The classic example is the loved one who asks after a relative who has died; for example, "Where's my mother?" Instead of stating the truth that the mother died decades ago, how much kinder it would be to skirt the issue and say something like, "Oh, tell me about your mother. She sounds like a wonderful woman!" Deflect and redirect. If you tell the truth that their mother has passed away, they may grieve as if it's the first time they heard the news. And to repeat that truth to them over and over again would be beyond cruel.

You may feel that you couldn't lie to your family member, but really, isn't it better to be kind? There are creative ways to not lie. Take the question about someone that has died. My first example was to redirect, but you could say, if your loved one believes in an afterlife, "Oh, she's having a great time now! You'll see her later." The questioning may repeat, but if you keep reassuring your loved one, she will feel heard.

❧

PRACTICE

1. Below are some scenarios that I would like for you to respond to—first with a correct answer, then with a kind answer. After you do that, think about some of the frustrating statements, comments, or questions that your family member makes and try out some creative, kinder responses.

    •   Bob wants to visit his daughter, but she moved from the area to another state some months ago. How would you respond to his question about wanting to see her now?

- Rochelle has always been a great dresser. Recently, though, her clothing choices have been more "creative." How would you answer when she asks, "How do I look?"
- Sarah loves sweets, but you know it's not healthy for her to eat cookies and candy all day. How would you respond to her repeated requests for another cookie?

2. Write the word kindness on several sticky notes and place one in each room of your house and on the dash of your car as a reminder to yourself.

Who Is on Your Team?

A wise, insightful friend asked me, early on in the journey, "Who is on your team?" I tend to be a lone wolf, a consummate introvert; I am used to figuring things out for myself. And doing it all myself. Isn't it a sign of weakness to ask for help? I am a strong person. I got this! So when he asked me this question, I hesitated and asked, "Team?"

"Yes, who are the people you can call on to help you navigate the waves that are coming?"

"Well, my parents, my sister, but I don't think I can ask friends to help out!"

"Well, think about it. You would help a friend in the same situation if she asked you." I didn't give it much thought after that initial discussion, but that question kept coming back to me, and over time, I did assemble a team, my village.

I started with professionals. I didn't initially think of them as members of my team, but that's exactly what they were. Knowing I needed help managing our investments and future expenses, I interviewed two financial advisers and chose one. He helped me gather all this information in one place and developed a plan going forward. I projected that I thought

Harvey would need in-home care in about five years, so I asked the financial adviser to outline a plan where I could retire at that time. He said that it was possible, and I rested easy knowing that was a possibility. Our children would be going to college in the ensuing one to three years, so a plan to pay for that was developed. I ended up not retiring, but maintained the practice and eventually sold it to an area hospital to become a salaried physician, and the financial planner held my hand through that process as well.

When Harvey's care needs exceeded the combined income from his disability checks and my salary, I engaged a lawyer who specializes in elder law. She outlined a plan to protect my assets if our savings took too large a hit. Harvey and I had established wills and powers of attorney, and living wills, so we met again with that estate lawyer to make sure everything was in order going forward. Our accountant helped me navigate the tax implications over the years of transitions.

Being a physician and caring for patients with depression and anxiety, I knew the importance of counseling and preserving good mental health. I can't count the number of times I have recommended that to a patient, but I had never seen the need for counseling myself. My life to this point had seemed charmed: my marriage was always secure; our children had had no behavioral or emotional issues. However, I knew that I would need a professional therapist to help shepherd me safely through the next years. I had friends and family that would listen to me and support me, but they loved me and were invested in my well-being. There is great value in finding a counselor who can be objective about a situation and not be emotionally involved in the one seeking help. I knew exactly who that person would be: Stewart, the chaplain from our college years, who also happened to perform Harvey's and my wedding ceremony. (Stewart once corrected me that he hadn't married us; we married each other!) It was Stewart who asked me who was on my team and forced me to think about loosening my grip on independence.

At our first session, as I described my perfectly balanced life that had become upset by Harvey's diagnosis, it was Stewart who observed that I would need to learn how to keep my balance in the midst of mounting waves. I would need to learn how to surf these waves and stay afloat. I have since seen this analogy in other settings, most recently at a physician well-being conference. The presenter showed a slide of roiling ocean swells, making the point that modern medicine can feel like this at times. She then showed a slide of a pier being ripped apart by waves, then a slide of a surfer gracefully gliding on waves. "Which picture do you resonate with? Wouldn't you rather ride the waves than be destroyed by them?"

In addition to Stewart and my legal and financial consultants, other professionals—Harvey's primary care physician, his neurologist, and later, social workers, nursing home directors, paid caregivers, and certified nursing assistants—were all critical persons on my caregiving team.

With my team of professionals lined up, I felt more secure. However, as Harvey's disease progressed, I did indeed need more help than I was able to provide alone. And Harvey needed more people in his life than just me! My parents live in our city, and I knew they would help if I asked. They loved Harvey and felt his loss acutely. They were there for me as a sounding board from the beginning. When I began attending an Alzheimer's disease support group, the location just one block from my parents' house, Harvey and I would eat dinner with them, then Harvey would stay with them while I went to the meeting. Most helpful of all was my father's willingness to step in whenever I needed someone at the house to supervise plumbing, electrical, or appliance work. I can't count the number of times I called on him to act as my representative while I was at work. We had two major plumbing disasters, and I had to replace two air conditioner units and a furnace. Obviously, Harvey couldn't manage these tasks, and I had to work, so my father became my surrogate in these instances. It really made me much more sympathetic toward single people who had to manage their home ownership alone.

When Harvey enrolled in a drug study, part of that study included a weekly four-hour infusion that could be done at home. Since I had to work, I fretted to my friend Hanna about taking this much time off. It wasn't my intention to ask for help, but she immediately volunteered to sit with Harvey during those mornings.

Another friend, Bill, heard that I was contemplating resigning from playing the keyboard in our church's band, something I dearly loved to do. It was becoming increasingly difficult at this point in Harvey's disease process to leave him alone for even just a few minutes because he would sometimes wander off. He would come with me to practice, but I couldn't be sure that he would sit and listen to the entire rehearsal. Bill said that he would gladly be with Harvey during these practices so that I could continue to play, essentially becoming Harvey's shepherd during those early Sunday mornings.

As more and more friends volunteered to help me when I expressed some concern or issue, it became easier to ask for help. Because I knew that we both needed social interactions beyond each other, I started asking friends to join us for a dinner out. Previously, we had occasionally gone out to eat with others, but rarely, so this was an opportunity for me to stretch our friend group a little larger. The guys in this enlarged circle of friends then started a weekly bowling group, expressly for Harvey, but without letting him know that.

Two different neighbors volunteered to walk dogs with Harvey. Our dog Nash, a beautiful collie, was beloved by Harv, but over time, Harvey would forget to walk him regularly, and these neighbors noticed their absence on the street and asked if they could walk together. We worked out a schedule, and at least three times a week Harvey and Nash would join either Jenny and Lily or Brian and Reggie in walks in the neighborhood or at a nearby trail. Harvey never met a dog that he didn't want to pet, and he became fast buddies with these two new canine friends, especially Lily, a black Labrador puppy that grew into an enormously social dog. This relationship between Harvey and Lily would play a large role in rescuing my husband one day.

For my exercise time, I would sometimes drive to a nearby gym first thing in the morning, while Harvey was still asleep, to get in a workout. I would return home, shower, wake Harvey, then eat breakfast and leave for work. One morning, when I returned from the gym, Harvey was not home. I called his name and searched throughout the house and the yard but could not find him. The cars were still in the garage, and Nash was in the yard, so I knew that Harvey had not taken him for a walk. My level of panic was increasing exponentially as I got in the car to drive around the neighborhood, taking his familiar walking routes, to look for him. I stopped any person I saw on the street walking or bicycling, and asked if they had seen my husband. I was truly frantic. He had never wandered off like this before, but of course I knew that it was always a possibility with dementia patients.

When my search was fruitless, I decided I needed to call the police, so I drove back home. I remember telling the dispatcher who took my call, "I'm not sure if you guys think this is an emergency, but my husband has Alzheimer's and has wondered off."

"Yes, ma'am, we definitely consider that an emergency. Has he done this before?"

"No."

"Well, I need to ask you some questions, then we will send someone out to look for him."

She then asked me to describe Harvey's physical attributes, what he was wearing, if he had any other medical issues, and a host of other questions that I considered so irrelevant at the time that I can't remember what they were now. She concluded by saying that I needed to stay at the house and wait for the officer to arrive. I was not to go out looking for him again. Argh! It was excruciating! I felt panic, terror, and guilt all at the same time. And where the hell was he?

No one would be looking for him until the police came and talked with me first. While I was gathering a photo of Harvey and looking through his clothes for clues as to what he might be wearing, I noticed his glasses were still on the top of his dresser. He was wandering blindly, literally! I couldn't just sit at the house waiting, so I decided to call Jenny and tell her what had happened and ask if it was possible for her to look for Harvey in the neighborhood while I waited for the police. She readily agreed, asking her husband to join her. I told her what areas I had already searched, so they went in a different direction and location. And found him, about a mile from the house! When they pulled alongside him, asking if they could give him a ride home, he refused, saying that he was fine, he was just out for a walk. When they couldn't persuade him, Jenny got out of the car and produced the enticement he needed—Lily! When he saw Lily, Harvey lit up, went to her, and began to pet her and talk to her. From there, it was easy for Jenny to get him into the car, with Lily to keep him occupied in the back seat for the ride home.

❧

Your team of caregiving help will become invaluable, even if you don't have one now or think you don't need one. I promise. Think beyond your and your loved one's usual friend group. Are there folks out there who are especially kind and caring that might step up to be on your team just because they are that sort of person? One surprising team member of mine was an old friend of Harvey's. They were best friends in college; Harvey was the best man at Chris's wedding, but through the years they had drifted apart, as old friendships can do. With Harvey's diagnosis, I knew that Chris would want to know about it, even if nothing came of it. Through Dennis, I tracked Chris down and explained the situation. He and his wife were living in Louisiana, but he immediately expressed a desire to come visit Harvey and me. That first visit was an amazing reconnection for them both, and after we arranged for two other college friends to join them, the four friends reminisced and shared old photos and just enjoyed being in each other's company. In the ensuing years, Chris and his wife would visit us, and Harvey and I visited them as well; it was a rich and wonderful experience for us all.

People that you think might be great additions to your team might not end up being so, or your team may change with time. Circumstances change for people, difficult situations can intimidate usually thoughtful persons, and someone who seemed like an ideal candidate might not be up to the challenge. We had two friends that I initially thought would be great companions for Harvey or support for me. I was disappointed when these two fell by the wayside, but I had to realize it was beyond my control and I couldn't force a relationship when the other person didn't want it. Though it didn't happen to me, family members that you think should be on your team can sometimes turn out to be toxic. You've heard stories of the long-distance sibling who just doesn't understand that anything is wrong with Dad. Or the other sibling who says it's too difficult for him to see his mother "like that." You don't need these people on your team if they wouldn't even want to play on the *same* team as you.

Your team will be invaluable to you. My team of professionals guided me through uncertain waters with sage advice. My family and friends gave support and companionship beyond the tangible help they provided. Because I was losing my confidant and best friend to dementia, it felt as if I had no one to confide in. Harvey didn't want to talk about his disease, even with me. This horrible thing was changing our lives, and I couldn't talk about it with the person I was closest to. My friend Nancy stepped into that void for and with me. She willingly became my sounding board when I needed to make a difficult decision, and guided me with wisdom that I couldn't see for myself, as I was too close to the situation to see a solution.

✍

PRACTICE

1. Make a list of your current team members. Now, think beyond that list. Who might you need to include that you hadn't thought of? Are there acquaintances that might be considered? Or old friends and distant relatives? These folks may not actually become a part of your team, but make a list anyway and expand the possibilities.
2. On a sheet of paper, list your particular skills and strengths as a caregiver. For each of your team members, list their skills and strengths. Are there any overlaps? Or holes that need to be filled in the future?
3. Think of a slogan or mascot or name of your village or team. Imagine designing a T-shirt that members would wear.

It's OK to Accept and Ask for Help

As I've mentioned, cooking was one of the chores that Harvey and I divided equally, the one at home being responsible for creating dinner for the one at the office. We each liked to cook and try out different recipes, though of course we had our favorite go-to dinners. For Harvey, it was "chicken under a brick" (but without the brick), grilled pork chops, and salmon with pesto. Whoever was not the cook on a given night became the dishwasher.

Once Harvey retired from practicing medicine, he became the daily cook and enjoyed it at first. As time progressed, his Alzheimer's did as well of course, and it impacted his ability to cook. The first noticeable change was a diminishment in his repertoire, meaning there were fewer and fewer dishes that he prepared. I didn't feel comfortable giving him advice and direction; he was still quite prideful and would take any suggestion I made as a slight upon his abilities. He might ask me what I wanted for dinner on a particular night, and I would have to answer with one of his favorites. Christina was still at home, now in high school, and I would occasionally ask her to help her dad with dinner, but I really didn't want to burden her with more tasks. She already had to deal with a father who was far changed from the one she had known.

Eventually, Harvey was unable to follow a recipe and would rely on his memory and instincts to create his old favorites. Dinners became quite interesting. Now, when he asked what I wanted for dinner, I knew that it was because he just couldn't come up with anything; his brain's file cabinet of recipes was not accessible. I would respond, again, with simple, favorite dishes such as black beans and rice, spaghetti with marinara sauce, or chili.

One memorable black beans and rice was very interestingly flavored. I have always prided myself on my ability to detect flavors in a dish, so I put my skill to the test with this one. The original recipe called for black beans in a sauce of honey, mustard, olive oil, and cumin. I could detect none of that, and when I asked Harvey what he had used, he could only answer, "Oh, this and that." I saw tiny bits of tomato or red pepper. Ah! That was salsa! But there was something else. I went to the refrigerator to see if I could get a clue. There it was! Worcestershire sauce. Black beans in a salsa and Worcestershire sauce. Gah! Not inedible, so I ate it and praised his creativity.

Another of his favorite recipes was tomato pesto, a simple dish requiring no heat to prepare, which used tomato paste, basil, olive oil, parmesan cheese, and garlic. When I suggested this recipe for dinner, he served unseasoned hot tomato paste over spaghetti noodles. I decided to take over the cooking after he served shrimp and grits. This was one of our all-time favorite recipes: shrimp sautéed in canned Italian tomatoes and bacon over grits made yummier with milk, butter, and cream cheese. Well, I asked for shrimp and grits, and that's what I got. Shrimp, still in their shells, stirred into a pot of plain grits. I was simultaneously giggling and cursing as I fished out the shrimp from their grits bath and tried to peel them. What a mess!

Once I took over the cooking, I had a variety of options to choose from. If there was a particular dish I wanted, and I was longing for some of my favorite dishes that were in my repertoire, I would ask Harvey to help me, giving him tasks like chopping or stirring. I would also pick up dinner from a restaurant on my way home from work, or pick up a prepared dish that only needed to be heated up. I found tasty frozen dinners at the grocery store that were quick to prepare, and I steamed vegetables and cut fruit to round out the meal. Then I had an idea to hire a chef to come to the house and cook with Harvey, providing companionship and giving him a purpose and a way to contribute to our household. It would need to be the right person, though, preferably someone who knew us and could relate to Harvey with ease.

When I told our friend Nancy about my idea to hire a chef, she said that she would do it. Now, Nancy would be the first to tell you that she is no chef; she doesn't really even cook. So I was surprised at her offer and asked her to explain what she envisioned this would look like. She said that I shouldn't worry about it, that she would come once a week to cook with Harvey, and that's all I needed to know. What she did was show up every week with a bag full of groceries, some recipes, and indeed cook with Harvey. She also brought along a blank spiral-bound scrapbook in which she placed copies of the recipes she used, the menu, and notes about their adventures that day. That scrapbook is one of my treasures now. Nancy even recruited another friend, Jill, a renowned cook who once studied in France, to cook with Harvey.

Jill showed up twice a month, also with a bag of groceries and recipes, which she added to our scrapbook, and she and Harvey would create marvelous meals together. His main jobs were to open cans (we had a rather unique can opener that no one but members of our household could operate), chop vegetables, and stir. Jill credits Harvey to this day with enhancing her original ice cream dessert recipe by adding copious amounts of chocolate syrup. Both Nancy and Jill continued their cooking sessions for a year and a half, finally stopping when Jill said that Harvey could no longer stir. I didn't know what she meant. How could he not know how to stir? She said that he couldn't incorporate with his stirring, and would instead just lightly rotate the spoon on the top of the sauce.

When I told friends about the amazing things Nancy and Jill were doing, another friend, Hilary, offered to coordinate some meals to be brought to us. Using an app that allowed people to sign up, and sending it to our shared friends' email list, she was able to have at least one other meal per week delivered to us. It was amazing!

Miraculously, right at the time "Cooking with Harv" ceased, a sign appeared on my driveway! While taking the trash out, I noticed a green credit card–shaped item lying on the ground. It was a coupon for HelloFresh. I had no idea what this was, but the coupon said it was good for three free meals if I used the accompanying code. So I looked it up online and discovered the marvelous world of home-delivery meal kits. I signed up right away, using the coupon code, and came home one day to a box on our front porch that held three individual boxes of premeasured ingredients and recipe cards. Each of the boxes held all the items needed to create a meal for two persons. No more measuring, as all of the spices were packaged in individual wrappers. No more spices on the shelf losing their flavor over time. No more wasted vegetables withering in my refrigerator when I didn't use them quickly enough. And my grocery bill plummeted. I have been a steady, loyal customer since 2014. That little green credit card coupon on my driveway was manna from heaven!

ᴄ⁄ᴐ

My story doesn't illustrate my point very well that you should be willing to ask for help! Indeed, I did not ask for help in the meal department, but you can! What I did learn was that I could accept help graciously and be very grateful for it all. In the previous chapter, I listed several other ways people offered to assist me, and that gave me the courage to ask Jenny and her dog, Lily, for help when Harvey wandered off. I don't remember asking for much other help, though. Instead, it felt like I had a multitude of friends wanting to help us and other friends that channeled their organizational skills to make it all happen gracefully.

As you think about asking for help, try to remember that people do want to help. It may be hard for you to ask for help, especially help with tasks you have always done for yourself. Your friends and family, your team, love you and your family member and probably have some of the same feelings you have about your situation. They may be grieving the loss of the friend they knew or feeling sorrow for the way your life has been turned upside down. They don't know what to do. They don't know what you need. Unless you tell them. Many people will ask you, "What can I do to help you?" and most mean it sincerely. So think ahead about what kind of help you need now or might need in the future. Be prepared when someone asks what they can do for you by answering them with a specific, doable task. And just ask!

Some caregivers feel as if they are the only ones who could possibly care for their family member the "right" way. It's not that it's difficult to ask someone to help; it's difficult to step aside and let someone else take the reins. I have seen this play out numerous times when working with a family in my medical practice. Usually with an older couple, the caregiver just cannot imagine letting anyone else care for their spouse, even for a few minutes so that they can slip away to the grocery store or hair salon. They feel as if no one could possibly understand their spouse's needs the way they can, and that's probably true, but unnecessary. What is necessary is time for one's self and one's own needs. It's OK to ask for help. It's OK to accept help.

Ↄↄ

PRACTICE

1. Think about what kind of help you need right now. Is it help watching your family member? Is it help with getting your loved one out of the house to socialize? Is it help with housework? Driving to appointments? Now look over your list of team members and potential team members. Who could you ask to help with this task? Don't dismiss someone because you think they wouldn't want to do that particular task. You don't know unless you ask. Don't hide behind the wish to be in control. Just ask!

2. On index cards, list several situations you are dreading. For example, maybe your family member is currently driving, but there will come a time when she can't. Or, in the future, your family member may not be able to toilet by themselves. On the back of each card, write the names of family, friends, or professionals who might help you. Hold each card in your hand and imagine a conversation in which you are asking for help.

3. Write the words *Ask for Help* at the top of your weekly or monthly calendar.

Put On Your Own Oxygen Mask First

When Harvey was diagnosed with Alzheimer's disease, I knew that my world would radically change. I was now a full-time physician running a solo practice. My previously well-balanced lifestyle was upended. The many outside interests I had developed and cherished were going to have to take a back seat as my new life shifted. Having worked part-time for all of my career, I had had the time to explore and create. The right and left halves of my brain were fully engaged. How was I going to keep sane without these life-giving activities? Would I have time to read, play the piano, study subjects outside of medicine, visit with friends, travel, or spend time in my art studio? These things had brought immeasurable meaning, purpose, and depth to my life. Was I going to have to drop them?

As I said in an earlier chapter, one of the first things I did was to start regular counseling sessions with a trusted therapist. I saw Stewart every month for nine years. This is not because I was a wreck and needed strength to navigate the waves, though that is surely a very good reason to enlist the aid of a counselor. My reason was more to be proactive, to know my next appointment with Stewart was less than a month away. He was another sounding board for me as well, like Nancy, a stand-in for the person I usually counted on for that function, my husband. Stewart did offer innumerable insights, some of which I am sharing here. It always helps to have an unbiased listening ear.

I joined an Alzheimer's support group about two years into Harvey's disease. I wish I had joined earlier, but I mistakenly thought I didn't *need* it. Maybe I didn't need it, but I grew to realize how important it was to my well-being. This group provided complete understanding, thoughts about new ways to tackle a problem at home, and a glimpse into what the future might look like. We were there for each other along the way. There were caregivers of spouses, parents, grandparents, and siblings, each with his or her own perspective. Under the leadership of our immensely beloved facilitator, Donna, we educated each other, offered different perspectives on a situation, and just listened. Each person was heard and held. We had deep, meaningful conversations about end-of-life care, when to start or stop certain medications, and the ins and outs of different living environments. I learned about geriatric psychiatry units, the difference between adult day care and respite care, and the difference between assisted living, specialized care assisted living, and skilled nursing. Sure, I could have read about all this, but the experiences of real people trying to navigate the care of their family members was invaluable. The group was ever changing as new people joined and family members passed away. We experienced people who showed up for one or two meetings, never to be seen again, and wondered aloud about what might have happened to one or another of them.

About three months after the Costa Rica trip, I realized that I needed to write down what was happening to my husband, myself, and our family. I wanted a record of events, but also a place to cry out my sorrow and anger. Because I had never routinely journaled before, this was new to me, but I couldn't ignore the pull to write it down. Filling six journals, I have a complete record of what we have been through. Yes, it's been invaluable in writing this book, but more than that, it's comforted me to know that our journey has been made tangible within the pages of my journals. (Did you catch that? *Journal* and *journey* are from the same root word.) When I read earlier entries, it takes me back to how I was feeling about the events of the time, bringing back memories and emotions that might be easier to forget, but were well earned and deserving of recognition. Yes, it's painful to read some of those entries, and I frequently have to put it down to cry, but there's healing in tears and memory. And as I said before, I couldn't pour my heart out to my soul mate, Harvey, because he refused to talk about it, and so I poured it out to my journals.

Reading has always been a passion for me. I distinctly remember getting back to reading after giving birth to my first child a year earlier. I had been too tired and busy to read during her first year, and I forgot how much I loved to read until I picked up a book and remembered. With Harvey's illness and the demands it made on my emotional state as well as the demands of a full-time medical practice, I just didn't have the mental energy to read. I had been in a book club for over six years when Harvey was diagnosed, and I didn't want to give up these treasured friends. They were very understanding on those occasions that I couldn't finish or even start that month's book. Someone suggested audiobooks as a way for me to "read," and I immediately became a believer and proselyte for the medium. I started listening to novels, memoirs, and the occasional nonfiction books in my car on the way to work and home again. I gave up reading, but I didn't have to give up literature.

I've already spoken about how I was able to continue to play the keyboard at church because of the kindness of our friend Bill as he shepherded Harvey during my band practices. I have a piano at home as well, and dearly love to sit and play for my own enjoyment and relaxation. Harvey always liked to hear me play, but I wanted my playing to have more of a connection with him, so I bought music books containing songs he knew and loved, and we sang them together: songs by Billy Joel, James Taylor, and the Beatles. Playing in the church band had pushed me, solely a sheet music–reading piano player, to learn how to play with only a lead sheet, a single page of lyrics with chords written above the words. I had to learn theory where I once had counted on sight-reading. I still don't have a good enough ear to "jam" with the other musicians, but I learned a lot about how songs are crafted. Now, I enjoy improvising on the piano, noodling around on the keys, creating melodies and interesting harmonies. Harvey was a willing audience to my meanderings, always appreciative by saying, "You just made that up? That's amazing!"

We continued to attend church regularly. Joining when we were newly engaged, Harvey and I had made a home at our downtown church, traveling twenty minutes each way to attend services and Sunday school. Because it was his wish that no one treat him differently, we kept the diagnosis a secret at first. We told friends that Harvey had retired for "health reasons." Eventually, the burden of carrying that weight alone became too heavy for me, and I began to share our story. Harvey still wouldn't talk about it with anyone, so I made sure our friends understood that he wanted privacy. The church continued to treat him, and our family, as they always had. I eventually took on the role of guide and interpreter as the disease progressed and robbed him of meaningful speech. He would hold my hand

and sit with me, silently present. The community watched out for him too, freeing me to socialize alone at times. He even came to church one morning wearing pajamas because I could not convince him to change. Anyone else might have elected to skip church that week, but I needed my community there, and I knew that we would not be judged, so we went!

Travel has always been important to me, and to Harvey as well. Once his diagnosis was made, I knew we had to get busy marking off some of our bucket list vacations. It wasn't easy, but as a family, we rafted down the Colorado River in the Grand Canyon for a week, took an overnight train trip across the western United States, and had an amazing week in Belize. It took careful planning, a great travel agent, and flexibility on all our parts to pull these off, but it was worth it. My journals are full of the details of each trip. The vacation to Belize was taken four years into Harvey's disease, and it was quite difficult on many levels; it was the last big trip we took as a family. The next year, we rented a beach house on the Gulf of Mexico and just relaxed and ate and enjoyed being together. Harvey and I took a few shorter trips together to visit friends. My best tip for traveling with a family member who has dementia is to be aware of and use the family restrooms! They were a godsend to me in airports, at rest stops, and even in retail stores.

One harrowing adventure at a rest stop without a family bathroom brought it home. Harvey went into the men's room, but didn't come out! I had to ask a man, as he was entering, to look for my husband and guide him out to me. This older gentleman kindly did as I asked and told me that he found Harvey standing at the window, looking vaguely out, clearly at a loss for what he was to do. I guess I could have announced my presence and walked in to find him if there was no one around to ask for help.

I also took several mini vacations by myself, with one of our daughters, or with a friend, leaving Harvey in the care of someone else. As a confirmed introvert, I knew I needed time alone to process and recharge, and the small trips alone did just that. They also served to educate our daughters, if they stayed with their father, as to what life was like at home, as they would sometimes minimize my concerns about their father's behaviors, saying, "It can't be *that* bad, Mom."

Exercising was not something that I did naturally or consistently, but I knew its importance and strove to stay active. I walked and ran in our neighborhood in the early morning hours, and when it became too cold for me, I would use our treadmill or go to the area gym. To care for my aching neck and shoulders, I booked monthly massages. I continued to see my physician, dentist, and optometrist for regular checkups. We maintained a healthy diet and limited alcohol use.

It was important to me to spend good quality time with Harvey, and not just be his caregiver. We were a couple, and I wanted us to do our usual couple things as long as possible. We continued to go out to dinner for at least five years. We went to movies that I thought he could enjoy; even if he couldn't follow a plot, big bright musicals were still enjoyable. We watched TV together, laughing at the antics of Lucy Ricardo, Barney Fife, or Ray Barone or crying over the melodrama that is Hallmark television. We continued to visit our neighborhood coffee shop each Saturday morning, and I often wondered what our regular barista there thought about the silent man whose wife did all the talking and ordering. We made regular visits to his parents, when they were in their home, as well as later, when they were in a nursing home.

To create something visually beautiful or interesting brings me joy, and I have usually always had some art project in the works. From drawing, to quilting, to jewelry making, my projects changed, but there was always something to create. Prior to Harvey's diagnosis of Alzheimer's disease, I had spent about five years immersed in paper crafting, mainly using stamps and ink to create custom greeting cards. I enjoyed layering papers and embellishing with ribbon and found ephemera. We had a good-sized basement room that was used as a man cave for Harvey's football habit and for the girls' video games. I claimed a nook area with a large wooden desk, and filed away my paper collection and tools. My father crafted custom shelving for my stamps, and voilà, I had a studio. We moved the larger television into the den so that Harvey could watch his games while I contentedly shuffled my papers and created small, usable works of art to give away. As Harvey's disease progressed, though, I didn't want to leave him alone with only the TV to keep him company; I wanted us to be together. I needed a small, portable art form that I could do while we sat together watching our comedies and Hallmark movies, so I taught myself to knit and crochet.

Then I encountered Zentangle. My sister had introduced me to this particular style of drawing a few years earlier, and when a patient showed me a piece that she had created using the same technique, I realized this was exactly what I needed. According to Zentangle headquarters, "The Zentangle method is an easy-to-learn, relaxing, and fun way to create beautiful images by drawing structured patterns." Traditional Zentangle drawings are done with black ink on 3½ inch square white paper tiles and shaded with graphite. They are nonrepresentational, so there's no questioning your artwork as not looking like it's supposed to. We are not drawing ducks or cars or trees; we draw simple patterns using only straight, C-shaped, and S-shaped lines or circles. Studying the official Zentangle website, and purchasing an instructional kit, I was on my way. Now I was happily creating little works of art, sitting on the sofa, while watching television with my husband.

න

As caregivers, of course we need to take care of ourselves. If you don't care for yourself, you can't be an effective caregiver to your loved one. This includes taking care of your physical body. Don't neglect your own health for the sake of your family member. Eat well, exercise, make regular visits to your physician(s). Don't neglect your emotional and spiritual health. Look up support groups in your area, consider finding a counselor, or schedule regular visits with your clergyperson.

If all you do is give and give, without pausing for time to do something that brings you joy, you will become lost in your role of caregiver, losing your own individual identity. Caregiving is the most important role you have, and to be the best caregiver your family member deserves, you need to be your best self. You can't be your best self if you cut off parts of yourself that give you life and joy. It's easy to say, "I need to take care of myself," but very hard to put it into practice when the needs of your loved one are so pressing. It's an obvious observation, but difficult to execute, I know. All the same excuses that I discussed in the preceding chapter come into play again. How can I leave my wife to do something I love while she needs me? I can't ask someone to sit with my mother while I get a massage! How selfish of me! *Please, heed this call.* Take. Care. Of. Yourself.

૭

PRACTICE

1. Consider these questions for your journal: What is keeping you from making better decisions about your own physical well-being? Why are you skipping your own doctor visits, giving up on exercise, or eating whatever is easiest to consume

at the time? Are you squeamish about seeking professional emotional guidance? Why? What do you do now for self-care? How does it make you feel to engage in whatever it is that brings you meaning? Do you feel guilty? Fulfilled? Both at once? What does your heart miss for itself? What have you given up in order to care for your family member? Is there a way to bring it back, if altered somewhat to fit your immediate circumstances?

2. Place a book of short poems, hymns, or prayers by your bedside to read to yourself or aloud to your loved one. Savor the beauty of the words.

3. Stop to appreciate the bigger perspective of an open sky.

You'll Have to Address the Driving Issue Eventually

Harvey loved driving. He was a very careful driver, with no speeding tickets or other traffic violations. Ever. The designated driver for all our excursions, either around town or to a farther destination, Harvey always drove. He taught both daughters to drive, as his was the better temperament for that job! He took consummate care of our vehicles, keeping each one running smoothly for as long as they lasted, so that in the thirty-three years of our marriage, we each only owned five different cars.

With his diagnosis, I knew there would come a time that Harvey should no longer drive; I just didn't know when that would occur or what form the realization would take. I chose to let him continue to do all the driving, mainly so that I could observe his skills in order to know when I needed to make changes. Of course, at first, there was no discernable diminution of his abilities.

The first sign of a problem was about one year into his diagnosis. A hubcap on the car of our youngest daughter, Christina, had disappeared, and Harvey was to go to the dealer to purchase a new one. Only he never made it there; he just couldn't figure out where the dealership was. He called me while driving, and I offered directions from where he was located, and he stated that he understood what I was trying to convey, but he still couldn't get there. Then he drove to my office to see if I could help him again. I wrote out the directions as simply as I could, but then he kept asking why he was going to the dealership; what was he supposed to get? He must have driven around for hours, but he never made it there.

He later told me that he just drove around, desperately hoping that something would look familiar. At dinner that night, Christina asked about her hubcap, and her father said that he had been unable to find the dealership. She had no idea what an ordeal the day had been for him, and innocently asked why he hadn't been able to find it with the directions written out. Harvey began to quietly cry, causing Christina to cry as well because she was worried that her dad thought she was mad that he hadn't gotten her hubcap. Harvey left the table, went into our bedroom, and began to sob loudly, then quieted down. He stayed for a long time, long enough for me to explain to our daughter about his day. When he came back, long after dinner had been cleared, he said, "I hate this Alzheimer's!"

This disorientation continued and worsened over time. He self-limited his driving range when he drove alone, knowing that he might get lost. He began to ask directions of me while we were in the car together. Especially at night, with no visual cues to guide him, I would tell him where to turn and what lane he needed to be in. One night after eating dinner out with friends, Harvey was to drive us home. Once I got him onto the interstate, it was our usual driving path home. This time, however, he asked me at every exit, "Is this where we get off?"

"No, not yet. Keep going."

Passing a familiar interchange, he exclaimed, "Oh, I know where we are now."

"Yes, we get off on the next exit." I relaxed a bit, but he still almost missed it. Even on the exit ramp, he didn't know which direction to turn, and I had to patiently walk him through which lane to enter, when, and where to turn. From there I thought it would be smooth sailing; we were on our home turf. But he relied on me for each and every turn until we got to our house.

"Turn right here."

"Here?"

"Yes, now!"

He drove very slowly, coming to a crawl at each suburban intersection, waiting for me to tell him to drive straight through or turn.

Almost home, he said, "I have no idea where I am." He was really scared and agreed that he didn't want to drive at night anymore, relieving me of having to make that decision for him.

My reaction to this was to be eerily calm. I could detach and at the same time feel his fear and feel sorrow for him. I was glad that we didn't have to have a fight about night driving, but worried that he might not remember this evening's misadventure. He did, though, because emotional events like this stayed with him longer.

Harvey was still a very safe driver by day, stopping at stop signs and red lights appropriately, merging with ease, driving at posted speed limits, using his signals correctly. The getting lost still occurred occasionally, but seldom in a big way. One day it took him three hours to get home from church alone. I was out of town and wondered why he wasn't there when I got home. He could only tell me that he got lost, got pretty far out, and had to ask for directions a couple of times. When I asked if he would like OnStar for his car, he became defensive about me wanting to know where he was. Even his father, on their forays to visit his mother in the outlying nursing home, expressed concern over Harvey's sense of direction.

I eventually purchased a tracking device for his car and covertly stashed it in his glove box. It would alert me when he left the house, and I could follow his movements on my phone, seeing where he was going and if I needed to rescue him.

Besides the episode that I described earlier about his banking incident, there were two other occasions when I tracked him to the bank, then saw withdrawals being made on my banking app.

I only had to rescue him once. One day, in the late afternoon of my workday, I was alerted that Harvey had left the house. I tracked the car in real time to a shopping mall near our home. The car remained in that location for a couple of hours, so that when I left work, I went directly to the mall to try to find him. The GPS had located his car in a particular parking lot, but I couldn't find it, so I left, thinking Harvey must have returned home while I was traveling. As I was leaving, I spotted him walking outside the mall toward the lot where the GPS said the car was located, and I turned around and followed him.

When I caught up with him, I rolled down my window and asked, "Everything all right?"

"Well, I can't find my car!" He got in and we drove around the lot again, looking for the car that wasn't there. There are outside lots and underground lots at this mall, and Harvey said that it was in an outside lot, so we drove around all the outside lots and still couldn't find the car. Evidently, the GPS wasn't accurate enough to pinpoint a car in a particular parking lot. We then drove through the underground lots until we found it, on the opposite end of the mall from where the GPS located it and where I found him wandering. With Harvey following me—in rush hour, no less—we made it back home safely. But I was a wreck! What if something had happened to him? What if someone had picked him up? Was he even able to ask for help?

At this point, he wasn't able to operate a cell phone and would forget to carry it most days.

That evening our conversation about this event was a turning point of sorts, as it was the first time he admitted that he was scared and frustrated by his disease, saying, "I try and I try, but it just keeps getting worse."

My heart broke.

In the ensuing months, he drove less and less by himself, with me always tracking his location to ensure he got home safely. Christina got caught up in the drama at times, scaring her in the process. He once told her that the car wasn't acting right and he needed to test it, so she decided to go with him as he drove. She worked to persuade him not to leave on several occasions, and one morning, as she was leaving for school, he asked if she would lead him to the gym because he wasn't sure he could get there on his own. She agreed, but was tardy that day, and worried the rest of the day if he had made it home all right. And still, his actual driving skills were intact.

At three years in with the diagnosis, I decided Harvey's driving days needed to be over. I researched and found that UAB, the large teaching hospital where his neurologist was located, offered driving assessments through the department of occupational therapy. I could call and make an appointment, but I didn't want Harvey to know it was my suggestion. I thought it would go better if someone else told him he needed that assessment.

At Harvey's next neurology appointment, I pointedly asked, "How are we going to know when Harvey should stop driving?" hoping the neurologist would pick up on my cues and recommend a formal driving assessment. He did, and it was scheduled. My research had taught me that the assessment would be conducted in three stages: the first to determine the level of cognitive impairment, then a driving simulation game, and if the patient passed those two stages, a driving test on the roads would be scheduled. I didn't know what to expect with the first two stages and was prepared to schedule the road test, knowing he would fail that because he wouldn't be able to follow the verbal directions. He didn't get that far, because Harvey performed very poorly on the cognitive tests as well as the driving simulation. I was present for all of the testing, but had to excuse myself for a bathroom break while they were still doing the simulation testing.

When I returned, the occupational therapist was explaining to Harvey about a toy, Bop It!

What?!

I asked what I missed, and she replied that Harvey had not scored well enough on the simulation to be able to schedule the road test, and that for now, he needed to stop driving.

"So why are you showing him the Bop It! game?" I asked.

"I was just telling your husband that if he practices games like this, it will help his reaction times." Then she pulled up the AAA website and showed us their driving simulation games. "If you practice these games, Harvey, you could come back and retake our tests and maybe improve your score so that you can drive again."

WHAT?

She told him he couldn't drive, then dangled this hope in front of him? *He has dementia, lady! He's not going to improve his scores!* Luckily, Harvey was mostly confused by all the talk—I could tell he wasn't taking it in—and he never latched on to the hope that he could retake the test.

He did catch a glimmer of hope when I told him that he had an eye exam coming up, and he exclaimed, "That lady said I couldn't drive. Maybe if I get new glasses, I can drive again."

His vision was fine. He never drove again, and was sad about it, and even cried a time or two, especially when I sold his car. I didn't want the car sitting in the driveway, tempting him to drive again.

ℰ⁄෩

I certainly didn't do everything right. I'm chagrinned at how long I let Harvey continue to drive despite all the episodes of getting lost. It's a hard decision for sure, one most caregivers dread. My support group spent untold hours hashing out this topic each time it came up.

Driving with dementia may not be an issue for everyone with this diagnosis; a few patients recognize their limitations and willingly give up their keys. However, for most, and maybe especially for men, it will be a hot button topic. Driving is a powerful symbol of independence. Just remember the feelings you had when you got your driver's license. Taking that away from a person can be demoralizing, even if absolutely necessary. You should try to prepare yourself for the inevitable day when it becomes necessary to make that decision.

Laws differ from state to state about the legality of driving with a diagnosis of dementia. Until recently, California required a physician to report any person with a diagnosis of even mild dementia to the Department of Motor Vehicles. Some state laws are unclear, and some do not even address the issue at all. If a state requires that they be notified when a citizen has dementia, they may take differing actions. Some states automatically revoke a license, some require further testing, and some do nothing. Insurance companies may require you to report a loved one's diagnosis of dementia, although some do not.

In any event, the day will probably come when you will need to take the keys. There is a lot of information and guidance available about how you might do this most effectively, while minimizing the dignity lost by your family member. One good idea I found later was to draft a document early in the disease process with your loved one that outlines precisely what skills are needed to continue driving, and have him or her sign it. You could elicit the help of your family member's physician, lawyer, insurance broker, or a trusted law enforcement friend. As a physician, I don't mind in the least being the heavy for a family that asks me to tell their family member that they shouldn't drive—after I've listened carefully to what the family has observed. If all else fails, you will have to disable the car, hide the keys, or sell it.

And remember, this is just one more loss of autonomy for your loved one. A very symbolic one, of course, but he may also lose autonomy in monetary transactions, cooking, communicating for himself, lawn care, shopping, and eventually dressing and personal hygiene.

∞

PRACTICE

1. Research the laws in your state surrounding driving with a diagnosis of dementia. Research what your automobile insurance requires of you. In fact, just to be sure, notify your insurance agent as soon as possible to be sure you understand how coverage and liability might be affected.
2. Research tracking devices and OnStar, or use your smart phone apps for tracking.
3. Make a plan now. Consider drafting a plan together with your loved one and having them sign it. If that doesn't work, brainstorm now about how you will address the issue. What skills will they need to continue to drive? If you live apart from your loved one with dementia, the next time you visit, inspect her car for scratches and dents. Go for an outing together and have her drive so

that you can assess her skills. If you are scared for your safety when she's driving, she shouldn't be driving!

4. You should probably start by trying to have a calm discussion with your family member as soon as you have concerns about his or her driving abilities. Explain gently what you have observed and that you want them to be safe. Sometimes someone will respond to the idea that others on the road deserve to be safe too.

5. Who could you ask for help? Look into formal driving assessments in your area. Ask the physician early on if he or she would be willing to make the determination. Who else might you ask?

6. Research other transportation options for your family member. Public transportation may not be appropriate for someone with confusion, but it might work well for others. Taxis are an expensive option, and there may be a volunteer driving service in your area. Friends and family may be available.

7. If you are dragging your feet on making this decision—and I'm not trying to make you feel guilty (well, maybe I am)—consider how you would feel if your family member was injured in a car accident or caused someone else to be injured.

Keep Your Family Member Active: Physically, Mentally, and Socially

"Can you see him? Is that him? There, coming around the corner! What's his time? Does he look too tired?"

Harvey was a marathon runner, and we, his family, his greatest fans. We attended most of his races, and armed with homemade signs and our loudest voices, we followed his progress by mapping out the course and strategically placing ourselves at points along the route. He was an amazing runner, and we were so proud of him!

Harvey always said that he was the best cross-country runner on his high school basketball team, but he didn't really take to running regularly until we were in medical school. He would say that running and training for 10Ks was his outlet for the mental and physical stress of medical school. In those days, he and I would scoff at the marathon runners who ran the yearly race in Birmingham in mid-February. "Ha! Look at those crazy people running for twenty-six miles on an early February morning. Who would do that?!" We just couldn't imagine the allure or time required to pull off such a feat. He stuck to his three- or six-mile training runs through medical school and during residency.

I'm not sure what tempted him to try his first marathon; maybe it was the challenge of it. We were back in Birmingham, with a new practice and a new baby. Was this life more stressful than the years of medical school and residency that he needed more time outdoors? In any event, he trained for his first marathon, the same yearly marathon in mid-February, using training plans gleaned from *Runner's World* magazine. He trained by himself in our neighborhood, occasionally taking the family collie of that time, Miss Kyle, with him on shorter jaunts. I remember helping him train for that first marathon by meeting him at preplanned points along his route with water, sports drinks, and snacks. He would look miserable to me, salt encrusting his forehead as he stretched his cramping leg muscles. At the end of that first marathon, he was pitiful: throwing up, shivering, barely able to walk, supported between his father and a friend. It took him three days to recover, as he limped around the office on punished legs. But the bug had bitten; he was hooked.

Harvey eventually was invited to join a running group by a friend from church who ran long distances with a cadre of his co-workers, training together for marathons that they also ran together. He had never run with others before, and this group quickly became his social circle. One or another of them would plan runs for the week, usually very early in the morning and on Saturdays, then divide up stops along the way that the others volunteered to stash with drinks and energy bars. Harvey was inspired by this group, especially one member who had the nickname Hillmaster for his ability to sprint up the infamous hills in our area. This group of guys ran the yearly February marathon together, not as a pack, but individually, for about seven years. They even traveled to Chicago once to run the famed Chicago Marathon.

Eventually, Harvey surpassed even Hillmaster in speed and decided to train on his own. He kept perfecting his technique, trying different strides that he had researched, all in an effort to remain injury-free and fast. He researched training regimens, again, finding one that would allow maximum results with minimal wear on the body. Other than a few minor strains, the only real injury he sustained was on a trail run at a nearby state park. Tripping on a root near the end of the race, he cut open his upper lip. Fortunately, a surgeon friend was at the same race and offered to suture his lip for him at his office, which was close by. I was always very proud of him, but would tease him about all the research he would do on running.

"Really, Harvey! What's there to learn? I'll teach you how to run. All you do is put one foot in front of the other over and over again, then do it faster and faster!"

Of course, he was in amazing physical shape, with a resting heart rate in the forties. Evidently running distances is genetic, because both of our daughters now run, and Elena became the star of her junior high cross-country team. She even ran her first marathon, at age twenty-five, with an amazing time, to raise money for our local Alzheimer's nonprofit organization.

Harvey's marathon career took off when he started to train on his own. Not held back by the group, he could push himself to new limits. He used a training schedule that had him running at the high school track one day a week, doing sprints. Another day was for interval training, with set distances and set time goals, with rest breaks in between. The third day was for hill training, and Saturdays were for distances, all following a prearranged plan. Yes, he was gone for a long time on training Saturdays, and he would awake early in the morning for the weekday runs, but I never minded. We had learned to give each other space and time to develop our individual interests at this point in our marriage.

His times improved, and he eventually had a time that qualified him to run the Boston Marathon in 2009, a year before his Alzheimer's diagnosis. The Boston is run on a Monday, and we decided that he would go alone so that I could stay home and keep the practice open. This is the trip that Harvey asked me to help him make travel plans for with airline, hotel, and ground transportation. I declined, wanting him to make his own plans. This was *his* trip; he could schedule his own arrangements. In hindsight now, I see that his trepidation of this task was perhaps that first inkling of a cognitive problem. However, he made the plans, all went well, and the office staff and I were able to track his progress because he was equipped with a computer chip that allowed us to watch his times. He did remarkably well. Another aspect of Harvey's running was his consistency. His mile times along the way were identical. He was a machine.

Boston was his last marathon before the diagnosis of Alzheimer's was made. He continued to run, of course, but now he had the luxury of time and could fully concentrate on improving his speed. Harvey ran five more marathons after his diagnosis, fifteen in all. He actually placed third in a small marathon in Jackson, Mississippi, and took home prize money. My husband was a professional athlete! He came in second in his age group in an Atlanta marathon, despite forgetting to pack his hat, gloves, and tights and having to borrow Christina's items, which were designed for a hundred-pound runner. Harvey's personal best was in February 2011, just five months after he was diagnosed, with a time of three hours, thirteen minutes—a remarkable time for anyone at any age, but for someone with Alzheimer's disease? Amazing! He ran three more marathons after that one, but his times began to slip. I noticed that his running calendar, which he used to track his training schedule, was becoming less specific and more limited in its range. He was running the same routes, ones that he knew well, because venturing off those well-worn streets was becoming too difficult to manage.

The next to the last marathon took place in Nashville, the Rock 'n' Roll Country Music Marathon, complete with live bands along the way. He had run it three times in the past, and it was one of his favorite races. It's a huge race with more than thirty thousand runners. He assured me that he couldn't get lost; there are just too many people running, with guides and supporters along the way. The race is much larger than our local marathon, so our daughters and I couldn't station ourselves along the way to cheer him on, instead opting to go to the finish line and wait there after we dropped him off at the start. The mob at the finish line was huge, and I was extremely nervous that we wouldn't see him finish, losing him in the crowd. However, Christina spotted him and ran along the fencing that separated the runners from the spectators, keeping him in her sights while Elena and I made our way to the exit shoot. Cell phones managed to get us all back together safely.

There was nothing remarkable about his last marathon in Chattanooga, Tennessee. Because it was a smaller, more manageable-sized race, I thought this was a good one for him. His time was about ten minutes slower than his personal best. After that race in October 2012, he told me it was too cold to run, and he never ran again.

I purchased a treadmill for myself and the girls to use during the colder months. Harvey used it occasionally, but it eventually proved to be too complicated for him to operate on his own, so I would push the buttons as he directed me to make it go slower or faster. I went to the gym that Harvey was using, Anytime Fitness, just down the street, to ask how he was doing, and spoke to a personal trainer, Jenny. She told me that she had noticed that something was "off" with him, but that he was doing fine in the gym. She wasn't put off when I told her of his diagnosis, because her grandmother had Alzheimer's, and she felt a kinship with Harvey and agreed to keep an eye on him. I eventually asked her to come to the house to work one-on-one with him when he was no longer driving. This worked out really well; Jenny, now with the nickname "Jennytime Fitness," would bring hand weights and other equipment with her twice a week. She would also operate the treadmill. She noted some irregularities in his gait and added balance exercises and hand-eye coordination games such as catch, which I continued with him.

When the weather warmed up, I asked Harvey to walk with me for my morning exercise, and he happily agreed. As time went on, and I hired outside sitters, they too would walk the neighborhood with him. Even in the nursing home, he was a walker, striding up and down the halls.

Beyond physical activity, I felt it necessary to keep Harvey's mind and social life active as well. He initially played brain-training games on the computer, then word-search puzzles. I tried to find jigsaw puzzles for us to work together, but he wasn't interested. I talked about my day and the patients I had seen, asking his opinion on a case, just to engage his mind. As a caregiver, I feel like I failed in this regard, in keeping his mind active. To keep him engaged socially, I arranged meals out, walks with the dog, and visits with friends. We kept going on vacations. When I had to hire professional caregivers, I left instructions that I wasn't interested in hiring a "sitter"—I wanted to hire a "doer." The two women I eventually settled on were adept at taking him on outings to a park, the botanical gardens, the zoo, or out to eat. Respite care with CARES provided even further social and mental stimulation. (More about our caregivers and CARES later!)

‿

I wasn't a perfect caregiver in regard to keeping my husband active in all aspects of his life—no one can be, but I tried. I knew what was important to him, running, and tried to keep that going.

It's important that your loved one stay active physically, mentally, and socially. It's just good for the body and the soul. It's good for you, too, as a caregiver. Better still if you can find activities to do together that fit the bill. I know that all this togetherness can be draining, but your family member needs you to be involved in making sure these happen. (You just have to remember to take care of yourself as well, right?)

The only things that research have shown to be beneficial in warding off dementia are maintaining a healthy diet, establishing good exercise routines, keeping active socially, and keeping active mentally. When I pointed out to Harvey's neurologist that he had done all those things his entire life, the neurologist just said that perhaps if he hadn't done those, he may have gotten the disease at an earlier age. We just don't know in individual cases what it takes to stave off this diagnosis, but the consensus of the scientific community is that a healthy lifestyle means less chance of dementia. Not a guarantee, but a generality.

The literature also suggests that keeping a person with Alzheimer's disease active in these modes of living will increase their quality of life, even if it doesn't increase their lifespan. Take physical activity, for example. The longer a patient is able to walk and maintain balance, the less likely she will become bedbound for long periods. If a person can continue to make personal connections with those around him, the richer his life will be.

☙

PRACTICE

Think of one activity you can have your family member with
dementia do to:

1. Increase her physical activity
2. Increase his mental activity
3. Increase her social activity

Ideally, these would be activities that you could do
together, bringing enjoyment to each of you. Or these could
be activities a paid caregiver could do with your loved one.
Your team of villagers could be asked to step in with some of
these as well. Research what opportunities are available in
your community in places such as libraries, senior centers,
community centers, local churches, and parks.

Enter Their World

I learned about respite care from my great friend, Nancy. I was aware of adult day care, and had visited three local ones to see if this was an option for Harvey. When he was first diagnosed, I thought that I would eventually retire early to stay home with him and care for him. However, I came to realize that I loved being a physician, and I was even good at it. Why would I quit? So I searched out adult day care, and was sadly underwhelmed by what I saw. Staffing was just too slight to have much of an impact on the participants, and one place seemed to use the television as a sitter service. I just couldn't see Harvey being happy at a place like this.

Nancy's sister was actively involved as a volunteer at her church in another city with the first program of its kind in our state. The idea was to provide respite for caregivers, hence the name, while giving patients with dementia a rewarding space and time to be themselves. Most programs run several if not all weekdays, for about four hours a day, and provide a lunch. Staffed mostly by volunteers, it's sometimes impossible to tell who is the volunteer and who is the patient; they are all participants. As Nancy explained what her sister's church was doing, it became clear that we needed something like this in Birmingham. We knew the place of worship had to be big enough to provide enough volunteers as well as a usable space and a kitchen. While we pondered this idea, Nancy, ever gentle, suggested that it was time to bring in outside help for Harvey. It was now about four years into Harvey's disease, and he was home alone with only the television for company. Nancy and Jill were coming to cook with Harvey, and Jennytime Fitness was coming regularly, but Nancy thought it was not enough. She saw him and what his life was like during those cooking sessions better than I could. When I told the neurologist that Harvey was getting lost inside the house, he also recommended outside help.

I first tried to line up private help with people I knew personally, but one backed out and the other just wasn't a good fit. Then I engaged a service, which sent two different sitters to the house, alternating them. I met one of them only fleetingly, and Nancy the other, but we were impressed by them and thought it would work well. However, I called home one day, and a third woman answered. I called the service and asked who they had scheduled to come out—five different women, four of whom I had never heard of, were to be coming. Please, Harvey had Alzheimer's; he needed consistency! I requested they please send at most two different sitters, and they complied. I would leave projects for them to complete together: baking cookies or brownies, carving the Halloween pumpkin, going for a walk, working on a photo scrapbook. I thought all was going well until I got an invoice for one month that listed eight different women! I cancelled the service.

Right at this time, Birmingham's first respite care was set to open. Nancy and I had been trying to plant seeds with the churches we thought would be a good fit, and indeed, Harvey's neurologist mentioned that he had been in discussion with one of these churches. Our hopes soared. Then, at Harvey's next neurology appointment six months later, he told me that the area Jewish Family Services organization was hoping to start a program soon. Nancy contacted the social worker there in charge of the program and met with her. It sounded like a good fit, and they were happy to hear that Nancy wanted to volunteer and that Harvey would be ready to be one of their first participants. Moving quickly, I applied for him to be in the program, and he was interviewed and deemed a great fit for their program. Nancy and he were charter members of Birmingham's first respite care, Caring for Adults through Respite, Enrichment and Socialization (CARES), located just minutes from our home. Harvey and Nancy went to CARES twice a week, and Nancy became their volunteer of the year and their music therapist.

What Harvey got out of this program was immeasurable. First, he was just one of the guys. He wasn't labeled as a patient; he was a participant. He had social interactions with people who cared about him, and in fact, I am told that he was the volunteers' favorite participant. They probably say that about all the participants, but it's nice to know they cared for him as the individual that he was. The CARES program provided activities throughout the four hours the members were there, as well as serving them a hot lunch. Not all participants want to become involved in all of the activities; that's one reason they offer so many. Harvey in particular did not care for arts and crafts—never did, never would. This is when the volunteers noticed that he loved to work on his "paperwork," busily circling and underlining items on a printed sheet of paper. But he loved the therapy dog, and tolerated yoga and music.

Harvey's favorite activity at CARES was balloon volleyball. With the participants armed with a swim noodle, the object was to bat a balloon back and forth over a net strung across the activity room. The only rule was that you were to remain seated. Only, Harvey's competitive side didn't want to hear that. When a balloon came his way, he would jump up and spike it over the net to shrieks of cheers from both sides of the net and the volunteers. He was in his element. The people at CARES met him exactly where he was, entering his world without forcing him to try to enter theirs. Perfect!

Through this experience, I learned to do the same, in a more natural way than I had previously done. Instead of being embarrassed by the attention he would give to a stranger's dog while on a walk, I would kneel with him and talk with the dog too, then stand and introduce myself to the person on the other side of the leash. I didn't care if they thought it was strange behavior. I did this when he interacted with children at the park too. Knowing that parents would be justifiably anxious about a grown man waving and chattering to their child, I entered into that play as well, and engaged the parents, rarely having to explain that Harvey had dementia. We began to play more together when we were alone, bopping balloons around the living room or dancing to a song on the radio, silly things that we had not ever done as responsible grown-ups!

I remember at breakfast one day Harvey pointed out the window excitedly and exclaimed, "Look at that!"

I couldn't see what he was pointing at from my vantage point, so I got up to look through his line of vision.

"Do you see it now?" he asked.

"No. What are you looking at?"

"That, there. See? It's moving now."

I didn't see anything: no bird, no squirrel. What was he looking at? Then I noticed the blinds move, and Harvey exclaimed again, "There, did you see that?!"

"The blinds? Are you looking at the blinds?"

"I don't know what they are, but they are here and they are there. Both."

My goodness, what in the world? Suddenly it clicked; he was seeing the reflection of the blinds in the window and was fascinated by the doubling he saw.

I jiggled the blinds. "Like this?"

"Yes! That's it! Isn't it great?!"

I had entered his world, a world of wonder and play. I learned to carry on "conversations" with him when real conversation was meaningless, just phrases and nods and smiles, but we connected over this shared time.

A few months after Harvey started going to CARES, I realized that he needed more one-on-one care than he was getting. Actually, it was Nancy again who said that she thought he needed someone with him at all times now. She was seeing what he could and could not do. He now seemed lost when I came home from work and would greet me with "Oh, thank goodness you're home!"

And I was finding all sorts of clues that he was just wandering around the house trying to find something to do. One day I came home to find a large packing box filled with random objects: boots, an iPod, bank statements, three sweaters, and several rolls of quarters. Another day I found him wearing an undershirt, three button-down shirts, two sweaters, a jacket, a hat, and one glove.

"Are you cold, Harvey?"

"No. Are you?"

He needed more care than CARES alone could give.

Nancy volunteered to look for and interview individuals that could be with Harvey throughout the day while I was at work. I thought we could use two people to cover from 6:00 a.m. until 6:00 p.m. This would give me time to walk alone in the morning, go to work, and relieve them when I got home. I had two names from people in my support group, so Nancy called them, interviewing them by phone, then arranged for them to come to the house to meet Harvey and me.

Linda did not work out so well! She and Harvey clashed immediately, as she was the hovering type, telling him what to do and when to do it. You just couldn't do that with Harvey. She lasted less than a week, when one morning Harvey had had enough of her and took off out of the house and down the street. Linda couldn't keep up with him and just shouted his name over and over, demanding that he come back. I couldn't answer my phone immediately when she called, so she phoned Nancy, who was vacationing in Belize. Dear Nancy called me, and I answered. She told me the story, then I called our neighbor Jenny, who got in her car with Lily again and intercepted him. Harvey happily got in the car with Lily, but Linda refused to get in the car with a dog, so she walked to the house while Jenny, Harvey, and Lily followed behind in the car. When they reached home, Harvey went inside, but Linda refused to follow him, staying outside talking with Jenny. I then sent one of my office staff to the house to retrieve Harvey and bring him to the office. Linda was still outside talking to Jenny. She resigned via text an hour later.

Caroline, however, slipped into our family's life seamlessly. Harvey was under her spell immediately, as she gently asked him to help her with chores rather than directing him to do something. She took him on an outing the first day, and as time went on, she continued to take him places—to shop for produce, out to eat for lunch, and even visiting with his mother at the nursing home. She also helped with daily personal care, such as assisting him with showering. She was exactly who Harvey needed in his life. Caroline even picked up on the exercises that Jennytime Fitness was doing and carried them on into every day. She also took him to the gym and ran the treadmill for him. She would then take him to CARES as her shift ended. Nancy then found SchRonda through contacts at CARES, and we were mostly covered. SchRonda had many years of experience with dementia and also slipped easily into our lives.

Our eldest daughter, Elena, had graduated from college at this point and had returned to Birmingham with a full-time job. Her boyfriend, Brett, decided to spend the summer in Birmingham, but found only a part-time job. I offered him a position as one of Harvey's caregivers, and he accepted. Brett would pick up Harvey from CARES and stay with him for the rest of the afternoon, playing basketball, running on a trail, even cooking a HelloFresh meal together. All three of these caregivers were more companions than sitters. They instinctively knew how to enter Harvey's world. And Harvey was happy and content in their care. I believe he thought of them as friends. His life was so much richer and fuller than it had been.

છ૭

A person with Alzheimer's or other forms of dementia cannot function in your world; you have to enter their world. In the 1980s the school of thought most espoused for caregiving was to reorient a patient to reality. Caregivers were instructed to correct their family members, trying to make sure their loved ones understood their world clearly. "No, you can't go home, your home was destroyed by fire in the 1960s." "Mother, you know I am your daughter, not your aunt. I'm your daughter. You can remember that." "Dad, you can't drive. Remember, the doctor said it wasn't safe." These are all examples of reorienting the person with dementia. Not that the information is wrong, it's just impossible at some point in the disease for your family member to remember. The medical and caregiving community eventually came to understand that reorientation only led to frustration and anger. How much better to see things from the loved one's point of view. (Remember the lessons of "It's better to be kind than correct" or "He's not giving you a hard time, he's having a hard time.")

I discovered a remarkable Alzheimer's caregiving blog early in my internet researching. It was written by Bob DeMarco, who was a caregiver to his mother. Bob had amassed a wealth of articles full of wisdom about caregiving. One of his best pieces addressed this issue of entering their world. After months of frustration, trying to make his mother understand something or other, it clicked for him that it was impossible for her to function in the "real world." He coined the term "Alzheimer's world," and to get himself prepared to enter her world, would literally step to the left before interacting with her. The act of actually stepping to the left reminded him that he was entering Alzheimer's world and leaving the real world. This might not work for you, but it's worth a try.

I also found that I could no longer communicate with Harvey as I had in the past. I learned to simplify my language, shorten my sentences, and use easier vocabulary. When words didn't get through to him, I communicated with gestures. Rather than tell him where to locate an item, I would point or walk to the particular drawer or shelf and say, "It's in there." Show and don't tell. Also, try breaking down a task into its components, one step at a time. Don't use unnecessary words.

☙

PRACTICE

1. Try rewriting these three conversations in a way that a person with dementia could better understand.

- Honey, could you bring me my glasses? I left them in the side table last night while we were watching TV and just forgot to bring them upstairs with me when we went to bed. It seems like I am getting as forgetful as you. Not that you can help it, but it worries me when I forget things like that. (Now, if you were a person with dementia, wouldn't you be terribly perplexed by this string of words?)
- Dad, I need you to gather all the information the accountant asked for and leave it on the desk for us to go through together.
- Mom, it's time to take your shower. (A family member with dementia may not remember the steps to take to accomplish this task.)

2. Consider other ways to make your loved one's world easier to manage. Purchase simpler clocks and calendars. Use your local library for books written at a level she would enjoy.
3. Try actually stepping to the left before you interact with your family member!

Plan for the Future, Don't Wait for Disaster

Well-meaning friends and patients would sometimes ask, "How is Harvey? Is he getting better?" Oh, my! What part of *Alzheimer's disease* don't you understand? Alzheimer's is a progressive disease; it's just going to get worse, in every aspect of a patient's life, and of course it did with Harvey.

One of the tasks he took over when he retired was the laundry. I never trusted him with my "delicates," so I would wash them myself, but he did the rest. The first sign that something was amiss with the laundry job was a slight pink hue to the white sheets, so I began separating the whites from the colored clothes. Then I noticed that he would forget about a load and leave it sitting to mildew in the washing machine, so I would start the first load, set a loud alarm, and he took it from there. He would fold his clean laundry and put it away, but would leave mine and our daughters' strewn over our bed for me to fold and distribute. I switched from unscented detergent to a fragrant variety so that I could sniff for freshness and make sure he was using detergent. Then I noticed a slight blue tint to the white sheets. Watching him start a load one day, I noticed that he poured the thick blue detergent on top of the clothes and didn't bother to adjust the water level. It was an easy fix for me to rewash the blue clothes, then just keep the water level set at high.

One day, I came home from work to find some of my dirty clothes folded on top of the bed, stains clearly visible. I realized that he wasn't actually washing the clothes, but getting them out of the hamper, folding them, and putting them away still dirty. Recalling what had been in the hamper, I searched out those articles of clothing and sniffed them for freshness. Not a pleasant task, mind you, smelling underwear crotches! I hoped this was a one-time event, but it kept happening, so I emptied our hamper each evening into one of our daughters' bedroom hampers (out of sight, out of mind), and took over doing the laundry.

Making up the bed every day was another of Harvey's routine jobs after retirement, and he mostly did a fine job with this until about three years into the disease. I would occasionally find the comforter upside down, backward, or sideways. The most interesting times were after he had washed the sheets and tried to make up the entire bed, the layers laid down seemingly at random. One day I found the bed made, from bottom layer to top: comforter, fitted sheet, blanket, top sheet, with pillowcases covering the decorative pillows. I thought the comforter was lost or misplaced, but there it was, under the fitted sheet.

Dressing himself also became progressively difficult. I've mentioned coming home to see him wearing multiple layers of clothing. He continued to wear long pants and long-sleeved shirts throughout the hottest parts of our summers. He began to wear the same clothes every day, putting on the prior day's clothes after his daily shower, sometimes even putting slacks on over his pajama pants. I began to gather up his dirty clothes when he was showering, take them to our daughter's hamper, and then lay out a clean set. Because white clothing blended in with our white bedspread, Harvey couldn't see it and would skip the underwear; I learned to lay out the white garments on top of our green blanket at the foot of the bed. I also learned to lay out the clothes in a stack in the order they should be put on; for example, underwear on top of pants, shirt on top of a sweater.

Then he began to have difficulty with certain items of clothing, but only sporadically. I found him once trying to put a sweatshirt on as if it were a pair of pants, one leg in each arm. Another time, he tried to put a pair of underwear on over his head, each arm through a leg hole. Each time, I would gently help correct the mistake, Harvey transitioning from confused to grateful as we sorted it out. I eventually gave up on getting him into pajamas at night. I moved to having him wear only elasticized pants—so much easier for the caregivers and me to assist him with. Button-up shirts and slip-on shoes became the norm.

He was able to maintain his personal grooming habits for quite a long time, though I did catch him trying to use the TV remote as a razor on his stubble, and Christina found him washing his armpits with soap and water at the kitchen sink. Eventually, he was unable to use his electric toothbrush, but could automatically brush with a manual one if I placed it in his hand. As time progressed, even that was too difficult, and he would just stand there with the toothbrush in his hand, looking confused.

I've mentioned that the family dog, Nash, was really Harvey's dog. The girls and I were not very good pet owners, but Harvey loved our dogs! With his retirement, Harvey took long walks with Nash and continued to feed and groom him. He had a routine for feeding Nash in the morning just as soon as we finished getting ready for the day. Then I began to have to remind him. During the winter months, and the especially hot summer, Nash spent the night in the garage, curled up on the patch of carpet at the foot of the stairs into the house or sprawled out on the cool concrete floor. So the first step of feeding him was to bring him from the garage to the fenced-in backyard, and eventually, Harvey and I divided the chore so that I set out the food while he brought Nash to the yard.

Nash was a very clever dog, and around this time, he started escaping out of the yard and wandering the neighborhood. He eventually settled into visiting two particular houses because the residents there were so friendly to him. I had a horrible time trying to figure out how he was escaping! I would find what I thought to be an opening under the fence, and block it, only to have him escape again. Harvey couldn't help retrieve him from the neighbors' houses, so it fell to me or Christina. Being in charge of Nash was the last item of managing the household that I eventually shouldered alone.

Five years into his disease, Harvey didn't remember he had a dog, and then Nash developed degenerative myelopathy, or as I renamed it, "doggy Lou Gehrig's disease." He had been dragging one back paw, then lost the ability to use his hind legs intermittently, then permanently. The veterinarian said the disease could last a year, but it was four months. Toward the end, I would ask Harvey to carry Nash into the yard in the morning and back inside at night as his ambulation deteriorated. One morning, I noticed he had not moved an iota from his spot at the foot of the stairs and called the vet to schedule euthanasia. But before I could get him to his appointment, he died there, alone, at the foot of the stairs, causing me to feel much guilt. I had wanted Nash to be able to lie on the vet's table, with us petting and talking to him while the vet administered the appropriate drug. Instead, Christina and I had to roll his body into a blanket and lift him into the back of her car. Once we were ready, Harvey got into the car with us, and we drove to the vet. We never told him that Nash had passed away, and we were able to get the body into the vet's office without Harvey noticing anything. Though he would have loved to have another dog, I knew that the care for a new pet would fall squarely on my shoulders, and I decided that I just didn't need another living being to take care of. Harvey did continue to enjoy canine encounters at CARES, on neighborhood walks, and when visiting with friends.

It's difficult for me to describe Harvey's loss of language skills. He was always a quiet person, so in the beginning there were no glaring deficits. What I noticed first was a lack of gravity in our discussions. We had always enjoyed debating and discussing current events, books and movies, theology; but now our conversation was light and fluffy, of no consequence or seriousness. Over time, Harvey had more and more trouble expressing himself, and I was left to guess at his meaning by way of context and gestures. Sometimes it was just impossible to understand what he was trying to tell me. He lost nouns and could only use pronouns—"Look, they're going up there," or "I see him with it and it's not good." He began mixing up the sounds in words so that "blessing" became "sibling." His ability to understand spoken language declined, and I had to resort to pointing and miming when I tried to communicate. Fortunately, he never got overly frustrated with his inability to communicate and would just shrug when either I couldn't understand his words or he couldn't understand mine. We still communicated with touch, hugging and holding each other close.

And then there was the phase when Harvey discovered and became fascinated with, and somewhat confused by, his new best friend in the mirror! He could hold a five-minute dialogue with himself, all gibberish, but with obvious language sounds, phrasing, and gestures. It was really cute. I think he knew this wasn't quite right because he would laugh at himself. I could actually enter into these nonsensical conversations too, and Nancy told me that he would have these kinds of interactions with some of the participants at CARES, both of them gabbing away without making any sense at all. I think it brought a sense of community and socialization to them both.

Harvey became more restless. Unable or unwilling to sit in his recliner watching TV for long, he would get up and wander around the house. I began locking all the doors leading outside, and eventually, even all the bedroom and bathroom doors except ours. I should have thought to lock the office door earlier because that simple solution kept him out of all the important papers. On our weekly grocery visits, I began to have to watch him closely, as he wouldn't necessarily follow me; instead, he would look down or straight ahead and would miss me making a turn. I slowed down. I wondered if his brain couldn't process all the visual input he was getting if he was looking around in the store.

I started to see some more signs of visual-spatial loss. He started lifting his feet dramatically as he crossed over thresholds, after hesitating first. He did this on sidewalks too, stepping deliberately over the concrete's sections. He became very hesitant on stairways, always holding on to the handrail, and eventually he could not go down stairs if he was holding a large object and not able to see his feet. Playing catch deteriorated, as did his ability to get into or out of a car.

Toileting issues started to become a problem about four years into the disease. It started with Harvey not using toilet paper, so that about every other day, he would show me his soiled underwear, and I would rinse them out and get him a new pair. I realized why this was happening when I found stool in the toilet bowl, but without any paper. Sure enough, his pants that day were soiled. Then I started to find used toilet paper in the trash can, then balls of poop in the trash can. One morning I awoke to find feces in the bathtub. He would occasionally have an accident in the shower, and I would find him trying to stuff it down the drain. Eventually, he could not make the connection that an urge to defecate meant that he needed to find an appropriate place to toilet. We were outside weeding early one morning, and as I glanced to where Harvey was, I saw him squatting in the yard. The paid caregivers, Caroline and SchRonda, dealt with his defecating in odd locations when they came on board, and did so with aplomb. By six years in, Harvey was in adult diapers, which made it easier on me and the caregivers, but he would still reach inside to grab a ball of it to show us. Even Elena and Christina had to manage their father's bowel movements. I knew that bowel incontinence was a probability with Alzheimer's, but I had imagined only adult diapers would be needed and thought that I could manage that easily. I had changed baby diapers for years. I was a doctor—it wouldn't gross me out. But let me just state this clearly, "Grown man poop is not the same as baby poop!"

One evening while at a restaurant, Harvey left the table to use the restroom. The door was in my line of vision, and when another gentleman entered, I could clearly see Harvey standing at the sink, urinating into it. When another man left, I could see that he and Harvey were gesticulating heatedly with each other! He didn't mention it when he got back to the table, and neither did I.

Then he began to get up in the middle of the night to urinate—sometimes in the toilet, but also in the sink or the tub. One night I vaguely heard pee hitting a solid surface, but I was too sleepy to do anything about it. In the morning, I found the bath mat was saturated. Another night, I found him sitting on the edge of the bathtub, directing his stream onto the mat, and another night, he peed into his closet, saturating the carpet and his shoes. Urinating issues became a nightly occurrence. I bought a toilet light, a night-light device that adheres to an open toilet lid and has a motion sensor on it, so that when

Harvey entered the bathroom, the device triggered and shone a light directly into the toilet bowl. That worked for a little while, and I learned to close the closet door and shower door before bedtime.

This lasted several months, and it began to wear on my ability to sleep. I tried to sleep through the night and just clean up whatever I discovered in the morning, but sometimes it was impossible. Like the night I was vaguely aware of a "plop" sound, not the usual hiss of urine. I roused myself and found Harvey at the sink, poop in his hands, on the floor, in his pajama pants, on his socks. I got him cleaned up, but it was 4:00 a.m. and I was awake for the duration of the morning.

Our nights became increasingly difficult. With all the toileting issues, I was not sleeping soundly. However, it didn't seem to affect me during the day. One night, Harvey was up and down continuously, with no bathroom issues, just restlessness. Obviously I didn't sleep well, half-awake just listening, but I dreamed that the toilet was full of feces and wouldn't flush. In the dream, I got up when I heard the toilet having difficulty flushing and found mounds of poop, which I placed in a large purple bucket. I tossed and turned after that dream, convinced it was real, and tried to figure out how I was going to manage all that mess once I got up. I was so convinced that this was reality that I was shocked to find the toilet clean in the morning. This was my life now—dreaming poop dreams in my few snatches of sleep.

I learned from my support group that the number one reason a family member with dementia is placed in a care facility is incontinence. I was handling *that* fairly well, but the lack of sleep was getting to me. And that is the number two reason someone is placed. The sleep issue ramped up as Harvey began having difficulty finding his way back to the bed. He never left the bedroom, but would wander around, sometimes sitting in the recliner by our bed, sometimes on the bench at the end of the bed. When he did eventually make it back to the bed, he couldn't get himself situated correctly, and invariably his neck would be cocked in an odd angle or he would rest his head on the bedside table. Sometimes, he would walk back to the bed and pull the covers up as if he were making the bed, even pulling the comforter up over my head and placing the decorative pillows on top of me! I had to sleep, but I felt as if I were sleeping with one eye and one ear open. I had decided, and said to myself and to my support network, that if my sleep was disturbed so that I couldn't function well the next day at the office, I would have to place Harvey in a facility. But, remarkably, I continued to feel well during the day despite my terribly restless nights.

About this same time, showers became much more challenging; Harvey just couldn't understand what the caregivers or I were asking him to do, replying "OK" or "Why?" but not complying. I think he actually meant, "I don't understand what you're saying." I would direct him to take off each article of clothing, sometimes gently tugging on a piece to get him started. Once he was in the shower, I would pour shampoo onto his hand and that would sometimes trigger an automatic action of rubbing his head. However, if I attempted to put his hand on top of his head, he would swat me away or act as if I were hurting him. A handheld shower wand was very helpful in rinsing him off. If Caroline or SchRonda had a particularly hard time getting Harvey to shower or change clothes, they would call me and I would talk to him over the phone, telling him that his friends at CARES were waiting on him and that he needed to get cleaned up so that he could go.

One morning I got a call from Caroline that Harvey just wouldn't shower and had walked out the door and down the street. He had been leaning into the water to wet his head, but wouldn't step into the shower itself. He finally got so angry that he stormed out of the house, naked! Caroline grabbed his clothes and caught up with him at the mailbox. She convinced him to dress, and then they walked together around the block, but when he kept walking, she got into her car and followed him. He was no longer angry, but wouldn't get into the car. She called me, and I suggested she just keep following him. She also called Nancy, who was able to come help. Harvey was now about a mile from the house, so Nancy pulled her car into a neighbor's driveway, got out, and approached him, saying that she was there to take him to CARES. As he got into the car, he gasped at his reflection in the window, his hair all wild and crazy. At that point it was easy to get him back home and showered and on to CARES.

The restless nights and shower difficulties just got worse, of course. After one particularly bad night—I was up cleaning pee twice, and Harvey just wouldn't settle down—I was exhausted to the point of tears in the morning. So I asked SchRonda if she could spend the night with us on weekdays. She agreed, and I finally had beautiful restorative sleep. I actually cried with relief that first night when I went to Elena's old bedroom to sleep, knowing I would sleep through the night without interruption. SchRonda camped out in the recliner next to Harvey's place in the bed, getting up to help him in the restroom and get him situated back in bed.

But it was time to start looking at memory care facilities. I had reached my deal breaker moment—I wasn't functioning well on limited sleep.

છ૭

Incontinence and sleeplessness are the top reasons for placing a patient with dementia in a facility. I was naïve to think that I could handle incontinence. Actually, I had envisioned Harvey wearing an adult diaper, and thought all that was needed was to change the diaper routinely. Incontinence per se was not the problem; it was the loss of the cognitive skills required to know what to do when the urge to defecate or urinate presented themselves. I hadn't foreseen that. He could be in a diaper, but he could easily pull it down to squat or aim! I was also quite naïve about showering. I had earlier thought that it would never become a problem for him because Harvey had always loved showers, taking two a day frequently. But, again, the cognitive losses made it impossible for him to remember the steps involved, and this set up his resistance to our care.

I never had to deal with a major disaster, and because I had decided ahead of time what my deal breaker was—my inability to sleep—I made a plan to look at facilities.

From my dementia support group, and through reading, I knew of several instances of a disaster occurring, and immediate placement had to be found. Falling and breaking a bone, wandering and becoming lost for a significant amount of time, physically lashing out at a caregiver and delivering unintended harm—I've heard all these stories, as have you. How much better to have a plan for that possible day. I recommend that you start looking at care facilities sooner rather than later. Even if you never use one, it is good to be prepared. Most allow you to pay a down payment to place your loved one on a waiting list. When his/her name rises to the top of the list, you can decide to take the spot or ask for a deferment. You may desire that your loved one stay in his/her home for the duration of the disease, but what if something tragic happens, and you haven't even looked into care facilities or other care alternatives? It's better to have an idea of what is available in your area.

の

PRACTICE

1. What is it that will force you to think about other care options for your family member? What can you manage at home by yourself or with caregivers? What is the deal breaker for you?
2. Look over the list of your village members and think about names or positions of people you may need to add in the future. You might have to be vague and simply list "someone who can . . ."
3. Write a letter to yourself a year from now. What are your hopes for yourself and your loved one? What wisdom has your future self gained? What new memories might your future self cherish?

"We Will Care for Him So That You Can Love Him"

S o I started looking at area care facilities for Harvey. I knew that he needed to be placed in a specialized memory care unit, called a Skilled Care Assisted Living Facility, or SCALF. I researched what was available, using a booklet called *Senior Living* that has franchises around the country, each franchise listing facilities in the area in graphs that include location, number of rooms, price, number of staff, etc. I also relied on my support group for recommendations for or against a facility, keeping in mind that just because one of their loved ones didn't do well in a certain facility, it didn't mean that Harvey would have the same difficulty.

I also used the services of a broker, an individual who had relationships with area facilities. This service was free to me, the broker receiving a payment from the facility where the client is ultimately placed. This broker met with me and detailed the facilities in our area, breaking them down into tiers based on cost. He also set up appointments for me and would accompany me to the facilities I chose to visit if I desired. I wasn't sure how much help he could offer me; I felt like I knew what I was doing, but I definitely see value for caregivers who feel lost and overwhelmed by the prospect. With the broker, Nancy, my sister, or one of our daughters, I started visiting the places closer to our home or my office.

I looked at a wide variety of facilities in terms of size, location, newness, and price. While I thought that a larger facility would rightly have more male residents, they just didn't feel like a good fit to me. There were too many residents, and I thought Harvey could become lost easily, and that it would be hard to keep track of him. Some of these large facilities were SCALFs only, with upward of ninety residents, and I worried that as the disease progressed, I would have to relocate him to a new, more highly skilled care nursing home. Maybe it would be better to find a facility that had multiple levels of care. Too small a facility was also problematic as there tended to be only one or two men there. Of course there were not many younger residents at any of these facilities, but when I spotted one, it made that facility more desirable to me. I guess I didn't want Harvey to be the only younger patient; maybe he would feel more comfortable if he weren't the only one. In reality, he probably wouldn't have known or cared, but it made me feel more comfortable.

I looked at three top-tier facilities and three middle-tier places. The lower-tier facilities were too far away for my comfort and ability to visit frequently.

The more expensive facilities were beautiful! Lovely manicured gardens, fireplaces in the common areas, and small intimate dining rooms were standard. At each of these places, though, we met with their marketing director, who gave us a tour of the facility, but didn't seem to understand dementia care. One of these marketing directors even asked a resident in her facility to recall her deceased husband's name! We saw few residents at these facilities, and I'm not sure why.

Therefore, there was little opportunity to watch interactions between staff and residents. These facilities also had sensory rooms, dedicated to housing equipment meant to help calm an agitated patient or stimulate a lethargic one. Unfortunately, the marketing directors knew nothing about this room and staff said they weren't ever used! They also had vignettes set up around the facility—small wall-mounted units dedicated to interests a resident might have. There were typically gardening, sports, kitchen, laundry, workshop, and military vignettes; but I saw no residents interacting with them, and one of my friends from my support group echoed that observation. The top-tier centers each had their own trademarked "care plans." In the end, I left these facilities impressed with how beautiful they were; I wouldn't mind living there! But. That was just the problem. It felt like they were developed to entice the patient's family, drawing on the family's need to place their loved one in a lovely facility. It was more for the family than for the one who would be living there.

I felt more comfortable with the middle-tier facilities. They certainly weren't as manicured or beautiful as the more expensive ones, and I had to learn to look through the cosmetics to see their worth. The marketing directors had more knowledge about dementia; I don't know why that is. One facility's director actually had a master of social work (MSW) degree and had worked in the field. Elena made this visit with me, and she was especially heartened by this woman's expertise with Alzheimer's. Another facility's marketing person readily admitted when she didn't know an answer to a question one of us asked, but immediately offered to take us to the unit and find someone there who could answer it. On the floors, we were able to observe interactions between staff and clients, most of which were appropriate and even endearing. When we were able to converse with the unit nurses, it became clear that they, too, "got it."

The last facility we toured was not on my broker's list. They didn't even have a marketing department; I had to call and speak with the unit coordinator directly to set up an appointment. When we met with Nicole, I found her to be calm and specific and not overly solicitous, factual but not cold. Her facility seemed to mirror her demeanor. It was almost serene, with a spacious and light-filled dining room, and the hallways were decorated with large, colorful photographs of local landmarks. Nicole was especially excited to show us their sensory room. She completely explained the concepts the room employed and demonstrated all the components. This facility housed about fifty patients, mostly older women, as I had come to expect, but there were about ten men and even one younger one. What clenched the deal for me was when Nicole said, "We will care for Harvey so that you can just love him." This was the one.

So about one month after I asked SchRonda to start staying overnight on weekdays, I wrote my deposit check and started the application process. Harvey had to have a physical exam, the facility needed to do their own assessment to see if he would be an appropriate resident, and I had to fill out reams of paperwork—including a complete financial statement.

I felt as if I was moving very fast, but Harvey's decline was proceeding rapidly. My plan to be slow and deliberate in choosing a facility was not an option. In the end, I went with my gut feeling, something I had done many years ago when choosing a college, a medical school, a residency program, and a practice location. Once the decision was made, I felt a deep peace. Fortunately, our daughters were on board with the decision as well, and we all moved forward in preparing for move-in day. Christina took her father to his primary care physician for a physical, and I shopped daily for items he would need and made decisions about which furniture he would take to the facility.

Nicole suggested that we move Harvey's belongings into his room over a weekend and move him in on a Tuesday. She wanted staff there to complete a thorough assessment and finalize a care plan over a four-day period, without family visiting during that time. So, we set a move-in date for about two weeks after giving the facility a deposit check.

A couple of incidents seemed to confirm my decision. I'm not usually one to put much stock in "signs," but these three offered reassurance when I was feeling especially vulnerable. It's a bit embarrassing to admit this, but I had actually asked God to give me a sign that I was doing the right thing. I knew it was silly, and I felt ridiculous saying it, even to myself. A week before move-in day, I made a big Target run. When I walked out of the store, right in front of me was a perfect rainbow. Not to the left or right, but flat in my face! "Thank you! I got it!"

Later that day, a Facebook memory popped up on my feed. It was a picture I had posted, a year earlier, of Harvey and me walking together, holding hands. I had captioned it, "When I hold his hand, he walks beside me, not behind me." I had meant it literally. When it popped up this time, however, I had the realization that maybe this is the relationship that God desires to have with us—to hold our hands and walk *with* us through life. I tend to walk ahead of God, forging and bulldozing my own way forward, up in front and by myself. I think, rather, that we are meant to walk with God and not rely solely on our own strength and will. Walking with God also translates into acknowledging that others can be the hands and feet of God by walking with us through life, just like all those beautiful souls who volunteered to help us did.

Another sign that the time was right to place Harvey in a good care facility came just before I signed the deposit check. Harvey had a grand mal seizure in the middle of the night. SchRonda screamed my name, awakening me from my sleep in Elena's old bedroom. I ran into his bedroom and found him on the floor seizing—all his limbs moving in a typical jerking fashion. It lasted about a minute longer, then he began deep rhythmic breathing and was completely unresponsive for about fifteen minutes. When he finally roused, he was very confused for another fifteen to twenty minutes.

I called EMS, and they transported him to the hospital. The evaluation there included lab work and a head CT, which required me singing to him to calm him during the process. During the six hours that we were in the emergency room, I had a chance to read about seizures in Alzheimer's patients. I learned that they occur in approximately 10–20 percent of all patients, and are even more prevalent in younger individuals and in later stages of the disease. I even learned that the average time of onset of seizures is about six years into the disease, exactly where Harvey was. Medications usually work very well in this population, so he was started on one. This incident really brought home to me that Harvey's decline was real; his seizure was a direct complication of his Alzheimer's disease. It was time he had more specialized care in a safe environment.

The weekend before Harvey's move solidified my decision; it was just too difficult for me and his paid caregivers, Caroline and SchRonda, to continue to care for him. That Friday night Harvey was up two to three times, but came back to bed fairly easily. Saturday morning, I needed to change his clothes but was met with total resistance to taking down his pants. I yanked them down to his ankles when the opportunity arose, then asked him to sit down. He planted his feet so firmly on the floor that I couldn't get the pants off. I tickled his right foot so that he lifted it, but he was so mad that he took off the pants and threw them at me. Then I had to rip off his Depends, and, placing a new pair inside a pair of clean slacks, I pulled up the combination of diaper and pants. Then came the challenge of putting on a shirt. The whole process took an hour; he would just shut down and become immobile when he felt forced to do these things.

While I was preparing Saturday's breakfast, Harvey wandered into the garage and defecated in a planter stored there. He napped in his recliner much of the day, then we visited with friends at their home for dinner. That went well except that Harvey wandered out of their house without any of us noticing. We found him in the yard, so he couldn't have been gone long.

Saturday night, he was up three times in the middle of the night, coming back to bed soon after. However, when he returned to bed at 4:00 a.m., I noticed that he had wet himself, the sheets, and the mattress pad. I let him sleep like that, but he was up and ready to go at 4:45, so of course I was up then too.

I tried to get him to shower; I even tried to entice him by getting naked into the shower myself, but it didn't work.

Then I began to launder the sheets and mattress pad, but Harvey sat his nasty, poop-smeared rear end on the mattress cover, and I had to launder that as well. When I turned from the washing machine, he was standing in front of me with a ball of feces in his hand and a puzzled look on his face. Unfortunately, I freaked out and screamed at him to put it in the toilet and wash his hands. Of course, he didn't understand what I was asking him to do; he just knew I was angry and reflected that emotion back to me. I had to forcibly wash his hands and his rear end, all while he was very angry, glaring and growling, but he never hit me. I understood that he felt violated by all this, but I just couldn't think of any other way to get him clean and clothed.

Now 7:00 a.m. Sunday morning, we ate breakfast and just relaxed, with me reading the newspaper and Harvey napping in his recliner. When he woke at 10:20 in good spirits, I decided we would go to church, but instead of going into the bathroom to urinate, he peed on the hallway table. We did make it to church on time, but I was nervous and anxious the whole time, holding on to his hand for the duration.

Next, we went to the grocery store as we always did on Sunday afternoons, but this time Harvey just couldn't follow my directions about where we needed to go for checkout and again when we were back in the parking lot. He was mad, and I was embarrassed—for the first time in my role as caregiver. Once home, he went straight to the bathroom and urinated on the closed toilet lid, then emerged with a small ball of poop in his hand. I overreacted again when he refused to wash his hands, and we fought, this time with Harvey grabbing my wrists and giving me fierce, angry looks. Eventually I just stormed out of the bathroom and went into the bedroom and sobbed.

Nancy texted me during my meltdown, and I told her what had transpired. She actually came right over and brought her iPod, loaded with seventies music. Music to calm the angry beast! She got him to wash his hands, then we all danced and sang together. His mood and mine were completely changed by this. When James Taylor's "You've Got a Friend" began to play, Harvey and I slow danced, and he tenderly kissed my forehead and cheek three times.

Nicole's words came back to me as we gently swayed to the song. "We will care for him so that you can just love him."

Once Harvey was placed in his new facility, I did indeed find it much easier to love him and leave the tasks of toileting and showering to the staff. Our visits were mostly calm and nurturing. When I arrived, he was overjoyed to see me, waving and grinning at me. If I left him to talk with the staff privately for a few minutes, when I returned, I got the same treatment from him! I often brought him his favorite foods to share. We danced or I sang, as music continued to connect us. Sometimes we would look through photo albums or picture books, or we would simply walk the halls, looking at the bright photographs or interacting with new friends. I played the piano for him and the other residents. When the weather was nice, we frequently went outside in their garden of raised beds, raised to waist level, actually, and walked or sat in the rocking chairs or watched the birds at the feeders. When I could observe him without him noticing, he seemed to enjoy interacting with the other residents, placing a friendly hand on a shoulder and nodding pleasantly in conversation.

Our departures from the facility ended up being quite easy. I would get him situated at the dining table and started on his meal, then we could slip out while he was occupied with eating. If it wasn't mealtime, I still found it was better not to say goodbye or tell him that I was leaving, as that brought on a long face and questions of "Why?" Instead, we would say, "See you soon!" or "We'll see you later."

Harvey was safe and content. As was I.

❧

Caregiving is hard, hard work, and it typically gets harder as the disease progresses. Care facilities do the hard work, often with great skill and hopefully with great empathy. They are trained professionals. Your loved one may never need care outside their home, and might never need professional caregivers in the home. But it is certainly important to gauge how well you are managing the task and to consider all your options.

❧

PRACTICE

1. Begin researching care facilities in your area. You need to know what is available. Consider working with a broker. What are the most important qualities to you in a facility? Ask friends and other contacts in your community who have transitioned loved ones into a memory care unit for advice and suggestions on possible problems to avoid.

2. If you are planning to place your loved one in a care facility, think carefully about how you will decorate and furnish the room. Some facilities are furnished, but some are not. You will want to create a familiar environment for her. It's also good to bring items that tell your loved one's story—diplomas, awards, photographs, and tools of her trade. Photographs from your family member's childhood as well as photos of her family of origin would be especially good to have. Your loved one will be comforted by being surrounded by familiar objects, and these items will also help tell the staff her life's story and just how amazing she is.

3. We found that bringing small gifts of food endeared us to some staff members. Be sure to praise and thank the staff for taking care of your family member. Kindness goes a long way. Try to visit your loved one at different times of the day and days of the week to meet as many different staff members as possible. If you visit at predictable times, you may only see the staff at their best.

4. If your visits feel overly long and frustrating, it's OK to shorten them to a manageable time that makes you feel good about the visit. How do you

say goodbye when you leave? Is there a better way
to do that if you or your loved one find it difficult
or emotional?

Imagine Waking Up in a Foreign Country and Someone Wants to Undress You

J ust two and a half weeks after Harvey moved into the memory care unit, I received a phone call from the nurse in his unit telling me that she was going to transfer him to a geriatric psychiatry unit. This floored me. He had been doing so well, adapting to the new space and new routine with aplomb. Or so I thought. The staff had not told me of any difficulties other than the ones I was having at home—resisting help with showers, wandering at night. Well, it was the wandering at night that got him in trouble. Evidently, he was more restless than usual one night and tried mightily to exit the building, eventually breaking the locking mechanism on the door. After that, the staff had a hard time getting him calmed down and said that they were actually scared for their safety.

I knew of geriatric psychiatry (geri-psych) units from members of my support group, but naïvely thought that it would never be a possibility for my dear, sweet, gentle Harvey. He just didn't have it in him to be an aggressive psychiatric patient.

So I pleaded for the nursing home to watch him for a little while, but to no avail. Then I asked if he could go to a particular unit that my support group seemed to like more than others. The nurse acquiesced to this request, but called me back to say that the unit only accepted patients over the age of sixty-five. A second unit in town was full, so he was sent to one about an hour away—actually, at the hospital with which Harvey and I had both started our careers. I knew most of the staff there, which was both potentially embarrassing and comforting.

I cancelled my afternoon appointments and drove to the hospital, meeting Nancy and both of our daughters there. Harvey had to be medically cleared through the emergency room before he could be accepted in the unit. I found him sitting upright on the gurney, looking like an overgrown toddler, clutching his blanket and stuffed dog, and grinning from ear to ear. Not the big scary man that broke down a door and supposedly terrorized the nursing home staff the night before! Part of the medical clearance required a urinalysis, only Harvey couldn't pee on demand, so the ER staff catheterized him. That experience transformed Harvey from a happy child into a confused, shell-shocked patient with dementia.

On the floor, the girls, Nancy, and I were oriented to the rules for visiting and met the staff and the overseeing psychiatrist. This physician outlined a plan to change Harvey's seizure medication from the one he was on, which the psychiatrist said was potentially more activating, to one that was more sedating. The hope was that this simple medication change would calm him and make his resistance to care more manageable. The psychiatrist also placed standing orders for Haldol, an antipsychotic medication that is usually used in schizophrenia, and Ativan, a tranquilizer, to use if Harvey became agitated while there. And he did. On the first three nights of his stay, he required injections of Haldol. Not that he was psychotic, but at low doses, it was being used to acutely calm this very agitated patient. Never in my wildest dreams would I have ever imagined my beautiful, kind-spirited husband would be given Haldol.

Harvey was in the geri-psych unit for twenty days, and was then released back to the nursing home. In order for that to happen, the nurse from his nursing home came to the unit to assess him again to see if his behaviors were better controlled. He was now calmer, but I could tell he was drugged—glassy eyed, with a hunched and shuffling walk, and very few words. He now had to be fed most of his meals, though he could occasionally feed himself finger foods. When we rolled him outside to the car in the required wheelchair, Harvey threw his arms wide open and exclaimed, "YES!"

Back at the nursing home, it took a couple of days for him to reacclimate, but he soon settled down, and we were told that he was doing much better, cooperating with showers and clothing changes. But I was a nervous wreck. What if he did something again and was sent back to the geri-psych unit? I doubted that the nursing home would take him back again. Then where would he go? Would any facility accept him? All I could do was check in frequently to make sure everything was going well. The nurse did tell me that Harvey was now more "touchy-feely" toward staff and residents, nothing sexual, just "handsy." Was this a problem? What's wrong with back rubs and pats on the hand? She was very vague about this possible concern, and just said they were watching that behavior for now. I noticed his gait became more fluid, he had better eye contact, he could feed himself again, and he was more alert and attentive.

On Thanksgivings, our recent tradition had been to eat dinner at the nursing home where his mother lived, meeting Dennis there. Their father had died two years earlier, and Lois was slowly sinking into her own dementia. Her nursing home was only five minutes from Harvey's, so I thought it would be a simple matter to load him up, eat Thanksgiving dinner, then head back for a longer visit with him. This day, Harvey had lots of trouble crossing thresholds and changes in the flooring, balking at each one, then lifting each foot high to carefully step over the demarcation. When we came to the edge of the sidewalk that butted up to the asphalt, he abruptly halted, and alarmed, shouted, "Water!" We convinced him it was safe, but then it took fifteen minutes to actually get him into the car. I made sure the child safety locks were secure, and we made it in time for lunch.

Harvey and his mother didn't interact much, but when he nodded off after lunch, Lois asked, "What's wrong with him? Is he OK?"

Then it was another fifteen minutes to get him back into the car and back to his place, where he promptly peed on the floor. Change and varying his routine usually brought on behaviors like this, so I vowed that our Thanksgiving lunches with Lois were over.

That next Monday, now one month since Harvey was back at the nursing home, his nurse called me to say they were going to have to transfer him to geri-psych again. I was stymied; I had been with him practically the whole long Thanksgiving weekend, and I had heard nothing from the staff that caused me to be concerned. She told me that she had been on vacation for the weekend, and that when she returned, she was told that Harvey had been wandering into other residents' rooms and wouldn't leave when asked. He had also grabbed a resident's shoulder and wouldn't let go; his hand had to be pried off. And he was peeing in public.

So off he went again, to a different geri-psych unit, this one about twenty minutes from home. Again, I met the psychiatrist and the nurses and learned this unit's particular rules. This time, the psychiatrist wanted to add Seroquel, which I had been expecting, as it is the medication most commonly used long-term to treat concerning behaviors in dementia patients. And again, his first two days there were very hard for Harvey. He tried to fight off staff needing to change his clothes and help him shower, requiring Haldol again.

Harvey was in this geri-psych unit for six very long weeks, through the Christmas holidays and beyond. We were allowed to bend the visitation rules on Christmas Day, so that instead of the allowed two visitors, the three of us were able to go together, bringing a new stuffed puppy as a gift. At this juncture, he had to be fed most meals, was walking with a pronounced lean to the right, and had lost most language. When the girls or I visited, we would sing Christmas carols, walk the halls while holding his hand, feed him a meal, or rub his back.

My most distinct visual memory of Harvey during this time was finding him in another patient's room, wearing one sock and carrying a shoe, completely lost and confused. I developed a repertoire of sorts for our interactions, partly as a way to gauge his abilities and also as a way to engage him. Sometimes he would dance with me down the hall as I sang, sometimes not. He could clap in rhythm to the song "If You're Happy and You Know It." My favorite times were when I could get him to imitate a pirate. Squeezing one eye shut, he would shake his head, and let out an "Arrrgh!" from the side of his mouth.

The prolonged six-week stay was because his nursing home refused to allow him to return. Adjustments were made to his medications, but mostly, the lengthy stay was spent trying to locate another facility that would accept him. This was the job of the social worker in the unit, and she assured me that they would not release Harvey until they found a suitable placement for him. She told me of some facilities that she thought would be appropriate, but they were all very far from my house and my office, so I asked her to check with places nearer to me. Two said that they were not equipped to handle Harvey's behaviors, another one was full, another only accepted patients over the

age of sixty-five, and another never returned the social worker's calls.

I knew of only one facility in town that had a behavioral
unit dedicated to patients with issues like Harvey's, and it
was close to my house, but a friend from my support group
had toured it for possible placement for her husband and was
extremely negative about it. (She actually had to place her husband in a facility in a neighboring state, as none in Alabama
would accept him.) Well, I had to see it for myself. If this was
the only facility that would accept him, I needed to investi-
gate it. Nancy actually visited and came back with a fairly good
impression, and I completely trusted her judgement. The marketing director who toured with Nancy even said, "If we can't
handle a particular patient's behavior here, they need to be in
the state's psychiatric hospital."

So I told the social worker that this was our first choice.
The paperwork went through, and we were set to go. The girls
and I decided to visit this facility as well, to see the place for
ourselves. When we met the same marketing person, she told
us that their intake nurse had assessed Harvey and said that he
would be a good candidate for their behavior unit. Great! So we
were shown the "Male Psychiatric Unit." It was horrifying! The
lights were dim, the paint was peeling from the walls, the floor
was sticky, and the odor of vomit and cigarettes permeated the
unit. I thought I was mentally prepared to see this unit because
I had experienced two different geri-psych floors of a hospital.
Nothing could have prepared me for this hellhole. As we left, I
asked the marketing director if this was the unit that she had
shown Nancy, because I was very surprised that Nancy would
have thought this was a good placement for Harvey. No. Nancy
was shown their two dementia units, not the behavioral unit.
Sheesh! We couldn't get out of there fast enough.

When I told the social worker at the geri-psych unit that
I would not place Harvey in this particular facility, she said

there were two more that might work. Both of them were far from my house, but at this point I did not care. One place turned him down, but hallelujah, the other one accepted him. It was a new dementia unit on a floor of an older nursing home. Nancy and the girls visited it first and reported that it seemed OK. It was very small, with only eleven to twelve patients but with room for twenty, and the staff seemed to understand how to work with patients like Harvey.

During these six weeks of trying to figure out where he could live, I wondered if I could possibly bring him home. I would have to hire two caregivers for parts of the day, and have around-the-clock coverage seven days a week. I wasn't sure if he could negotiate the stairs in our home, and there was no place for him to pace. I thought about adult day care, but he wouldn't be able to get into and out of a car twice a day. I thought about buying or renting a small one-level home for him and a care-giver, but I really couldn't afford that. The situation was just horrible, but there was nothing I could do about it. And it was even more horrible for Harvey. I felt like he had no quality of life left except for the brief pleasure of eating a meal. He wasn't really responding to us anymore. I even wrestled with a fantasy about slipping him some sort of medication to end his life, but the last thing our daughters needed was to have their mother in jail for murder.

Also in the midst of Harvey's lengthy geri-psych stay, I sold my practice to a large hospital in town and transitioned to become a paid employee and began using an electronic medi-cal record system. It was all months in coming, but the actual transition day fell squarely in the middle of that December.

Harvey moved into his second nursing home and actually did fairly well there. Nancy, Dennis, the girls, and I visited him regularly, bringing him chocolate treats and smoothies, walk-ing the short hallway, or going outside in the courtyard if the weather permitted. His unit was small, old, cramped, and with low ceilings. The smell here was an overbearing floral scent intended to cover fouler odors. He continued to resist care, but the staff learned techniques that worked with him. And Harvey continued to decline, losing the ability to clap to our song or do his pirate imitation. I felt like he recognized me as "his person" about 50 percent of the time, but he no longer recognized the girls. If asked, he still responded that his name was Harvey.

He was at this second nursing home for seven months before I got the dreaded call that he was being transferred to geri-psych again. This time, he had tightly gripped another resident's wrist, hard enough to draw blood with his fingernails. This was something we had noticed for some time. His grip was very strong, and he could grab hold of anything and not let go. Not in anger, but just as a baby holds firmly to an object, a grasp reflex. He just could not let go. The geri-psych unit that Harvey was sent to was yet another one, this time at the hospital closest to my house. As I had come to expect, on his first day there, he required an injection of Haldol, but he soon settled down. The psychiatrist here said that he just wanted to observe Harvey for about a week, but doubted that he would change any medications, especially when the nursing home confirmed that they would accept him back.

And two months later, I got the phone call again. "Well, he didn't really do anything. He just seems to be in the middle of most of our behavioral issues, even if he doesn't cause any harm. His medications need to be adjusted in a geri-psych unit so that he can be calmer."

"What? He didn't do anything, but you're sending him anyway?" I didn't say it quite that way, but the nurse would not back down, and followed through with the transfer.

I asked that he be sent to the unit in the hospital closest to my house again. He was, but the nurse hadn't called ahead, and when he got there, we were told that there were no beds available and he had to be transferred to a different unit.

I decided to use this hospitalization time to try to find another memory care unit that might accept him—one that was closer to home. It was almost a year since all the places in town had refused him, and he was no longer exhibiting the behaviors that they had previously objected to. Might as well try! Harvey was released back to the second nursing home after a week's stay at geri-psych, but transferred to his third and final nursing home shortly after. It just took longer than one week to make all the arrangements.

Harvey's final nursing home placement was to the facility where his parents had been. Lois was living on the floor below where Harvey would be, and we looked forward to having them visit together. The wing Harvey was assigned to was designed for more advanced dementia patients, those that needed a higher level of care than a typical memory care unit, but who were still ambulatory. The hallways were wide and long, the lights were bright, and his room was spacious. The unit's nurse had been employed there for seventeen years, and the activities director had been there for twenty. They understood the difference between resistance to care and aggressive behavior. They talked about redirecting and behavior modification, instead of medication, to control unwanted behaviors. Harvey became more alert and responsive, even pointing to a photo of his mother once and exclaiming, "Mother, that's my mother, mother!"

One month later, though, Harvey was back at geri-psych for the fifth time. This time, forgetting where his room was, he had climbed into bed with a female resident who fell when she was trying to get away from him. There was nothing sexual about the incident, but the facility worried about the appearance of such, and also had genuine concern about the safety of other residents if this behavior persisted. He was at geri-psych for observation for one week, then released back to the nursing home. But they would only allow him back if I provided sitters for one-on-one care for twelve hours a day—on top of the usual nursing home fees. I had no other options, and this plan worked! Having someone with him at all times kept Harvey out of trouble. The sitters could redirect him out of other residents' rooms, help feed him, and walk with him down the hallways, keeping him safe.

ॐ

The title of this chapter comes from a teaching point that had a huge impact on me. I can't remember when or where I heard this, but it has stuck with me as a way to explain resistance to care. Imagine yourself waking up every morning in a hotel in a foreign country where you don't know the language. Now imagine that a stranger walks into your room, and in the native language, tells you that he is there to give you a shower and change your clothes. As this stranger starts to disrobe you, what would you do? Of course you would lash out and fight against this indignity. Imagine now that you try to leave this hotel room, and you find all the exits are locked. Of course you would try all the locks, forcibly. If you couldn't get out, you'd pace and rant and walk into all the rooms that were open, looking for an exit. This is exactly what the person with dementia experiences each day. They are in a foreign land where they can't understand the language and strangers are doing things to them, and there is no way out. Of course they fight the care. Is it aggressive behavior? Or resistance to care?

It is beyond the scope of this book to discuss how to deal with such behaviors in detail. There are good resources available that detail ideas for getting your loved one bathed, dressed, toileted, and fed, their teeth brushed and hair combed. In general, it is agreed that you should approach your loved one slowly and from a face-first position, not from behind. Speak slowly and gently, using simple language. Break down the action needed one step at a time. For example, at some point in the disease, you can't simply ask a person with Alzheimer's to brush their teeth. You will have to place the toothpaste on the brush, place the brush in her hand, and direct her hand to her mouth. Try covering her hand with your own as you gently move the brush to her mouth; this makes her feel like she is the one moving the toothbrush. While you are doing this, explain what you are doing each step of the way. If that doesn't work, try another approach. And ask for help. And do some more research.

Truly aggressive behaviors that could harm another person certainly need to be addressed quickly. I have heard too many stories of caregivers that were pinched, hit, or squeezed to the point of real harm being done, and often these caregivers feel they are helpless to do anything.

Geri-psych units are different and separate from adult psychiatry units in that patients are older, either with psychiatric diagnoses, substance abuse issues, or dementia; or, like Harvey, they have a disease that is more common in older patients. I have a friend from my support group whose husband also had younger-onset Alzheimer's disease and was once admitted to a regular psychiatric unit. What a nightmare! Staff there didn't understand how dementia manifested itself and were chastising the poor man for "inappropriate behaviors" that are quite common in dementia, but he couldn't understand and change those behaviors. I counted it a blessing that some geri-psych units accepted younger patients and knew how to handle these behaviors.

The main goal of a stay in geri-psych is to monitor the patient, and, if necessary, adjust or add medications to safely control behaviors that cannot be tolerated in care facilities or at home—behaviors that are seen as dangerous to the patient, the staff, the caregivers, or other residents in care. It seems to necessarily set up a tension between two camps—the care facility desires quiet, calm clients (medicated, if necessary), and psychiatrists desire that patients be as alert and interactive as possible. Nursing homes are not allowed to administer medications such as Haldol on an as-needed basis, a term called *chemical restraint*, so the patient has to be well controlled on daily maintenance medications instead.

Unfortunately, there is no easy or simple approach to dealing with unwanted behaviors.

രാ

PRACTICE

1. If you are having a difficult time with a particular behavior, research different approaches to try, or discuss it with your support group or your loved one's physician.

2. Imagine yourself in the scenario I painted at the beginning of the previous section. Now, journal your experience as you lived it in your mind or make a drawing to represent the emotions you experienced.

3. Draw a map of the island that is the foreign country of Alzheimer's disease that you, your loved one, and family members inhabit. Use words and images to detail the places where *you* get lost, feel lonely, and don't know the language. Acknowledge your own sense of being lost and alone in a foreign country. How can you escape the island temporarily? What is your favorite spot there?

Acknowledge Your (Ambiguous) Grief

I began to grieve the loss of Harvey in my life as soon as I realized that he probably had Alzheimer's disease. I knew that there were many shared dreams and goals that we would never be able to realize. As the disease progressed, I lost more and more of him. The essence of Harvey, the flame of the divine within him, would never die; it was just harder and harder to see it embodied. I knew he was in there somewhere, but I was losing him.

Three reminders that his love for me still held firm occurred in the third, fourth, and sixth year of his diagnosis. In the first instance, Harvey and I were watching TV together in the den when he leaned over to me and with a smile on his lips and a slight gleam in his eye said, "Do you think we should get together?"

"We *are* together," I replied.

"No, I mean get together," he said as he intertwined his fingers together and nodded his head.

"Oh, do you mean we should get married?" I asked.

"Yes!"

"Well," I answered, with a grin and a lift of an eyebrow, "We *are* married! We've been married twenty-eight years. And we still love each other very much!"

"Oh, good," he said with a satisfied laugh.

About a year later, I walked into the den to find Harvey watching our wedding video. I had recently converted our VHS tapes to DVDs for us to watch together. One of our daughters had put in this DVD for him to watch, but he really didn't understand what it was.

"What are you watching, Harv?"

"This," he replied, while pointing to the TV. "I don't know what it is."

"Well, it's the movie of you and me getting married."

"We're married?"

"Yes, we've been married for twenty-nine years now and we love each other very much."

"Wow! I knew I liked you, but I didn't know we were married," he exclaimed with much joy.

The last episode occurred when he was newly moved into the first memory care unit. I was visiting and had the radio tuned to the seventies station. As "Landslide," by Fleetwood Mac, started to play, Harvey beckoned me to him, and with a gentle smile, enfolded me into his arms, and we swayed to the music.

Toward the end of Harvey's life, he began to laugh or giggle unexpectedly and uncontrollably. It was really quite cute, but we could never figure out what triggered it, even though we tried very hard to replicate it. When he started crying for no reason, it hit me. He was exhibiting signs of pseudobulbar affect, a condition that can occur in patients with neurologic disorders or brain injuries. The exact cause of this condition is unclear, but there is some type of dysregulation between a patient's true emotional state and the emotions they exhibit. It can be quite unnerving, especially if a patient laughs or cries at completely inappropriate times.

I, of course, had periods of deep grief, striking mostly in unsuspecting moments. My journals record my laments and sorrows along the way, and reading them now still brings up those emotions. A love song on the radio could bring me to tears, as could a particularly touching movie. I was struck numb when I watched older couples at the airport, heading off to a vacation together. I grieved at family gatherings, lost in the loss of Harvey's presence in future holidays and events.

At the beginning of this journey, I grieved especially so for our daughters. How would they manage in this world without their father? Then I would fall on my knees in grief if I allowed myself to imagine Alzheimer's disease befalling one of them. They both confessed to worrying about this possibility from the very earliest time. I sought to reassure them that they had the same chances of developing Alzheimer's at a young age as the general population, which is very low, but they countered with, "But so did Dad." We knew that both Harvey's parents had some form of dementia, and we did learn that Harvey himself had at least one gene for older-onset Alzheimer's disease. The girls weren't worried about getting the disease late in life; it was the younger-onset version that terrified them. And me. They asked me to have him tested genetically, to see if he carried any of the three known genes for younger-onset Alzheimer's disease. To be honest, I dragged my feet. I just didn't want to know if they stood a chance of getting this same horror. I didn't know if I could deal with the knowledge that Harvey might have passed on a gene like this. I did eventually get him tested, and he did not carry any of these genes. Unfortunately, this did not reassure the girls. If he didn't have the gene, then we didn't know why he got the disease, and that meant they could too.

Choosing a college was extremely difficult for them. I tried to keep my hands off their decision-making, and I think I succeeded. Harvey had been diagnosed at the start of Elena's senior year of high school. She had always known that she wanted to attend an out-of-state college, but now she worried that she should stay closer to her father. She was undecided between a college in a neighboring state, three hours away, and one in town, where she would live on campus. I knew that she preferred to move away, but she seemed to need my permission to do so. Without my telling her that I wanted her to choose the out-of-state college, she eventually knew that she had my blessing. She made her decision just before the deadline.

Prior to move-in day, she and I decided that just the two of us would load the cars and do the move ourselves. There would be too many people on campus, and we would need to socialize with her roommates and their parents. It would just be too much for Harvey; I would have to cover for him the entire weekend. I don't think he knew or cared this was happening without him, but I grieved for Elena, and for Harvey, that they weren't able to share that experience. Her four years at college were wonderful for her, as she fully immersed herself in the experience. She would have preferred to continue to live in a city away from home, but by the time she graduated, she felt pulled to return to Birmingham to be with her father for the time he had left.

When it was time for Christina to consider colleges, Harvey was four years into the disease. She looked at several colleges, some out of state, but in the end, felt that she needed to stay close to home, for her own sake. She chose to attend a college in Birmingham, actually the same one Harvey and I attended. She lived on campus, and also fully immersed herself in the college experience. Her move-in day was very hard for me. There was no possibility of Harvey going with us, and in fact, at this stage of his disease, I couldn't leave him alone.

Elena and Brett played the parental roles and moved Christina into her dormitory while I stayed home with Harvey. Later that day, after most other parents had left, he and I went to campus to see her and her dorm room. I cried many tears that day, realizing that I couldn't help my daughter move into college, and that I was now home alone with Harvey, with no one else to talk with. I had come to the stage in my life that I had dreaded. I had a giant baby bird in my empty nest.

Though Christina was on campus for four years, she continued to be integral to our family because she was in town. She always came when I called with one of Harvey's medical or psychiatric emergencies. He developed appendicitis five years in, and Christina met us at the hospital. When he had the seizure, she again came to the emergency room and stayed with us overnight, even though it was her birthday. She actually spent the night in the emergency room with her father while we waited for a bed in the geri-psych unit to open. What college student has to do that? I grieved deeply for her loss and added responsibilities. Through it all, she confided in her boyfriend, Phil, and very few friends, preferring to keep that part of her life private. I was proud that both girls recognized that they needed counseling and sought it out themselves while at college.

The most stressful time for me throughout Harvey's illness was when his behaviors were ramping up, and I had to make a decision about moving him into a memory care unit. It was then that a close family member told me that I had a bald spot. I assured him it was just my natural hair part, but when I looked closely, I had indeed developed a half-dollar area of complete balding at the crown of my head. Another area near my hairline then showed up, this one an area of extreme thinning, and with white hair. Both patches grew, and I had to ask my hairstylist to find a haircut and style that I could use to cover them. They did grow back in after about a year. Stress can indeed make your hair fall out!

I've mentioned that one of the conversations that Harvey and I used to love having was dreaming and scheming about selling our big family home and moving to another part of the city once our daughters had moved out. We had endless discussions about which neighborhoods we liked, and if we even wanted to live in a neighborhood. Maybe we would move to an area lake, or find a place on a stream. We could live anywhere we wanted, buying a smaller home and just enjoying getting to know each other again. That dream had to die. In any case, by the time Christina had moved to college, a big move like that would have totally disrupted Harvey's equilibrium.

Once Harvey moved to a nursing home, I got the itch to move. I was rambling around in our big house by myself, and it just felt nuts to keep doing that. Also, his care was expensive, and I reasoned that if I sold the house and moved to a smaller one, I would generate cash that could go toward his care. When he settled into the second nursing home, I began my search. It was a seller's market at the time, so my plan was to buy the perfect house as soon as I found one, then turn around and sell my big one. I knew my big house would sell quickly because of its location, and I wanted to take my time in finding a new one and not feel pressured to find one when the big house sold. I found a gem of a house in an old, established neighborhood, built in 1925 and just a little less than half the square footage of the big house. It was perfect. I put an offer on it the day it listed and moved in six weeks later. Harvey would have loved this new home.

The next step was to get our big house ready to sell. There was tons to do, but I made a list, and with tremendous help from my realtor, we knocked it out. (My sister was my realtor, actually! I was her first buyer and seller.) I decided what furniture and decor I wanted to take to the new house, and sold the rest in an estate sale. The big house sold the first day it was on the market, two months after I moved to the new house.

After that, the next project was to be Elena and Brett's wedding. (More about that in the next chapter!) Once the wedding was over, the holidays came and went, and then I crashed. In a one-and-a-half-year period, Harvey was in three different nursing homes and was admitted to geri-psych five times, and I sold my practice and became an employed physician, bought a new home, sold the old one, and hosted Elena and Brett's wedding. Of course I crashed! What in the world was I thinking by juggling all of those balls at the same time? Was I trying to distract myself from Harvey's reality? Maybe. Probably. And it worked. I was happy managing all the projects; I rarely felt overwhelmed by them at the time. And by crashing, I don't mean that I fell apart or quit working or somehow disintegrated. I continued to see my counselor and thought that I was processing all the changes fairly well. But grief caught up with me and came crashing over me like a wave, flipping the surfboard that I had been riding so competently.

Without the projects, I became very lonely and very sad. I felt trapped in a sadness that would never resolve. I couldn't move on with my life because Harvey was still alive. Alzheimer's has been called "the long goodbye," but at this juncture, it felt more like interminable grief.

Our church was starting a six-week grief support group, and I felt compelled to join it. However, I wasn't sure if this would be appropriate since my loved one was still alive, and all the other participants had lost theirs. I asked the facilitator if she thought it would be OK, so she asked the other group members, and got back to me to say it would be fine. This group was amazing. They completely accepted me where I was; I didn't have to explain that my grief was as valid as theirs, even if Harvey hadn't passed away. The group was eight in number, people from the ages of sixteen to eighty, male and female, who had lost husbands, wives, fathers, and mothers. One session's assignment was to tell the story of our loved one, using props if we wanted. I brought Harvey's Boston Marathon medal and his stethoscope and told the group all about this wonderful man. Each of the participants told their stories as well, and we celebrated the life of each of these souls. Another night, we were invited to bring a favorite food to share in a meal together, choosing something that our family member loved to cook or to eat. I brought Harvey's famous "chicken under a brick" (but without the brick), and we all ate, and then wrapped up our sessions together. It was very healing for me to share my grief with people who understood what I was feeling. I wasn't sure if I would need another grief group when Harvey actually died, because this one was so cleansing.

એઠ

Grief rarely comes to us wrapped neatly in the five stages described by Dr. Elisabeth Kübler-Ross. Yes, grief encompasses denial, anger, bargaining, depression, and acceptance, but they just don't present themselves in a logical progression. I experienced each of these stages multiple times, in all periods of Harvey's illness. I recognized I was grieving, but I didn't have the words to describe my grief at the time.

Our daughter, Elena, the social worker, introduced me to the term *ambiguous loss*. This is a term coined by Pauline Boss, a PhD psychologist whose work in the 1970s centered on the families of soldiers who were missing in action during the Vietnam War. They had no body to grieve, no closure. This type of loss lingers, with no resolution. Ambiguous loss may be a physical loss, such as a missing person, or it may be a psychological loss. This applies when the physical body is still present, but the person is psychologically absent, such as in traumatic brain injury or dementia. A person experiencing this type of loss may be the family of the patient or the person themselves. In both of these types of ambiguous losses, there can be no closure, and grief is unresolved. Dr. Boss's work also addresses the types of grief experienced by those living through ambiguous losses. Anticipatory grief is what I experienced during the eight long years of Harvey's illness. He hadn't passed away yet, but I knew what was coming, and I grieved each of his mental and psychological losses along the way. It helped me to label the type of loss and grief that I was experiencing; I felt validated by being able to name it.

୧୬

PRACTICE

1. Remember, you are grieving already. Are you someone who embraces sad feelings or runs from them? Pay attention to these inclinations and begin choosing moderation, or balance, in these two ways of approaching grief. A counselor or pastor may be of great benefit if you are feeling overwhelmed by grief.
2. Prepare your loved one's favorite meal, and celebrate who they were with people who love and support you. What other rituals might you employ to honor your grief?
3. How does your grief feel today? Gather dark markers or colored pencils and write, draw, or even scribble on a piece of paper. Then wad up the paper and place it in your pocket or purse for the day.

Let's Do It Together

Elena and Brett met in college, actually on the first day of Biology 101 his freshman year, her sophomore year. They became friends almost immediately, and over the course of that school year tentatively built a relationship. Elena told Brett about her father roughly halfway through the school year, bringing their relationship to a deeper, more vulnerable level. A few months after that, they were a couple. When Elena graduated, she moved back to Birmingham and rented a house with two other young women. As I've mentioned, Brett spent that summer in Birmingham too, completing an internship and working for me doing yard work and helping care for Harvey by picking him up after CARES and entertaining him until I got home from the office. After he graduated, he, too, settled in Birmingham with a job as a project manager for a company that pairs health coaches with clients seeking a more comprehensive approach to their health care needs.

On a weekend that I was away for some alone time, during the period when Harvey was up and down all night, Elena spent the night at the house with him. One morning, when she tried to get him showered, Harvey would have none of it. She called Brett, who came over, and together, while singing Bruce Springsteen songs to him, they got him showered, toileted, and clothed for the day. Actually, not together, but they tag-teamed with each other, so that when one of them got frustrated, the other would switch places. Brett had won his place in my heart and in our family.

A few months after that, Elena started dropping hints to me that they were thinking about getting married soon. Harvey was newly in the first nursing home, and Elena made it clear that she wanted to marry before her father passed away. She was feeling me out about the idea and wanted to know if I thought that they were too young.

"No," I said. "You're both mature, have good jobs, and are obviously committed to each other."

But I was conflicted. Was this a good reason to get married? And did I have the energy to help plan a wedding? What if we planned the wedding and something disastrous struck with Harvey? Would she want her father to be present? Was that even possible? And who knew in what shape he would be when the date came? It really didn't matter what I thought, of course; it was their decision, but I was a bit uncomfortable. Then I realized why I was mentally balking. It was forcing me to acknowledge another big loss of a dream. Harvey would not be able to walk his eldest daughter down the aisle, or dance with her in a father-daughter dance at the reception, or give the final toast. One more loss to mourn. It hurt, at a time that should be joyous.

Three months later, when Harvey was settled in the second nursing home, Brett asked if he could come to my house to do some yard work for me. Of course! During dinner, he told me that he was ready to ask Elena to marry him. He didn't ask my permission, thank God! My daughter is not my property to give; he just wanted me to know. I had been planning on letting Elena use my engagement ring as hers if she wanted, because I wasn't wearing it any longer, preferring to wear just my wedding band and an anniversary band. I told Brett this and offered to retrieve it. He was a little taken aback and asked if I was sure. I hadn't worn the ring since Harvey had given me the anniversary ring in 1995, so yes, it was fine with me. I was thrilled now that it was really happening.

But it took Brett two months to finally give the ring to Elena! They called me an hour or so afterward, and I invited them to come to my house. Christina and Brett's sister joined us for a bottle of wine and lots of pictures. They told us that they wanted the wedding to be in about six months, and got busy planning it right away. They secured our church for the ceremony and an event venue near my house for the reception. My worries about having the time and energy to help plan a wedding were unfounded; they did all of it themselves. My role was to be a listening ear for ideas and to affirm decisions made. I was thrilled when Elena asked me to walk her down the aisle and to give the final toast at the reception. The wedding planning proceeded without any hitches and with just a modicum of bridal anxiety.

The only concern was how to include Harvey. Elena initially insisted that she wanted her father present at the wedding, even if he couldn't walk her down the aisle, and said, "He would want to be there." The wedding was still six months away, and we didn't know in what shape he would be at that time. I didn't think it was a good idea to plan on his being there; we needed a plan B and a plan C if we couldn't pull it off. We discussed the idea that Elena, Brett, Christina, Phil, and I could go to the nursing home between the ceremony and the reception, taking a small celebration there. Or maybe the couple could visit with him the next day. She was going to have to be all right with whatever happened, and we were all going to have to be flexible.

When the month of the wedding came, we were still undecided about how to include Harvey. Elena and I knew that it wouldn't be possible for him to sit on a pew in the congregation, but she really wanted to see her father on her wedding day. I just couldn't see how I could make that happen. There would be too many things I needed to attend to that day, and I couldn't get to the nursing home to pick him up and then take him back. Once again, I forgot to ask for help, and Nancy showed up with the solution. She volunteered to transport Harvey to and from the church before the ceremony. I bought a new shirt, slacks, and belt for Harvey to wear and took them to the nursing home, then explained to the nurse what our plans were. They would let Nancy borrow a wheelchair, and she would get him into her car and to the bride's room at the church about an hour before the ceremony. If Harvey couldn't cooperate, and it was impossible for her to accomplish this task, we would accept that outcome, but we had to try.

One week before the wedding, Harvey was sent for one of his geri-psych admissions, the one for being in the middle of most of the nursing home's behavioral issues, a bogus reason for a transfer in my book. My pleading made no difference to the nurse's decision, even when I reminded her of the wedding plans. Elena called the nurse, and as shocking as it sounds, the nurse replied, "That is exactly why I didn't have a wedding. Too much drama!" Not a hint of sympathy for Elena, even implying that she was stupid for having a wedding.

Harvey landed at the geri-psych unit on a Friday, a week and a day before the wedding. Elena was lost in sorrow and not sure that she could go through with the wedding with so much sadness and anger and confusion. She should have been bubbling with happiness and excitement, but instead, she had to deal with her father's psychiatric stay as well as the possibility that he might not make it to the wedding. It was hard on all of us to try to handle these two events at the same time—the hospitalization and the wedding. I wanted her to focus on the wedding and let me worry about her father, but her happiness seemed to depend on whether or not Harvey could be present, even though she had prepared emotionally for that possibility. But how do you prepare emotionally for *this* reality? A psychiatric hospitalization is a far cry from Nancy not being able to get Harvey into her car. Elena and Brett's honeymoon was planned as a two-week trip overseas; now she was fearful of even leaving at this point. As the week progressed, she brightened somewhat when she had the realization that her father would want her to be happy and to concentrate on the wedding, not his situation. She acknowledged that it was hard for her to compartmentalize, but that she would have to.

Happily, Harvey was released from the hospital back to the nursing home on the day before the wedding, and we were back on track with the original plan. It all fell in place, and ended up being a lovely day, all of it. Nancy enlisted two more of our friends to help her with transporting Harvey to and from the church, and that ended up being absolutely necessary. The nursing home had administered his medications early, thinking that if he were more sedated, we would have an easier time with him. However, he was overmedicated, and could barely walk because of that, and Nancy and the two friends had to practically manhandle him into the church. Elena, though, didn't seem to notice because she was so full of joy for the day and for the gift of the presence of her father on her wedding day. We were able to share a beautiful time together as a family. Harvey, our daughters, our soon-to-be son-in-law, and I ate a small meal together, had our photos taken, then Nancy and the friends took him back.

As I walked her down the aisle, Elena carried a bouquet embellished with a charm she had made with a photo of her father. At the end of the aisle, we met Christina and Brett, who were waiting for us at the altar rail, and the four of us went to a small table we had set up earlier with a candle and a photo of Harvey. Elena lit the candle, and we walked back to the center of the altar. I hugged and kissed her, and lovingly squeezed Brett's hand, then left them at the altar together. The ceremony was fairly traditional; my mother, Elena's grandmother, read a passage of scripture and our pastor delivered a homily that focused on couples caring for each other through all of their lives together. I teared up when Elena and Brett read the vows they had both written to each other.

The reception was perfect—the weather, the venue, the food, the music, the dancing, the games. We had it all. In the dining area, we had set up a table to hold photos of all the family members who weren't able to attend—those who had passed away and those who had been unable to travel. Instead of wedding favors, Elena and Brett elected to donate the earmarked money to our local chapter of the Alzheimer's Foundation, placing that announcement on the same table.

I delivered my toast on the outdoor patio, where the dancing would later take place. I had memorized it, and was able to present it smoothly. Elena and Brett were standing right in front of me, both of them quietly crying as I spoke. I shed no tears during the toast, but I certainly did while composing it.

As a wedding gift to Elena, I wrote the following poem and gave it to her that day.

Dandelion

I remember sitting with my daughter
On a patch of scruffy lawn, grass and clover and weeds,
Leaning together as we blew the stars-on-stalks off a dandelion.
Watching down parachute away.

How singular that moment was,
Just the two of us, a usual day, a usual weed.

The soft prickliness of that perfect white sphere,
The translucent tiny globe, held us.
Watching down parachute away.

And I remember sitting as a family in an airless exam room,
She, now almost woman, he, the father-husband-patient.
"Will he one day forget who I am?"
Still as stones, we labored to breathe in the vacuum
That was left of our lives.

How singular that moment was,
The three of us stunned into silence,
Clutching the edges of our dreams
As they slipped away, like his memories will,
Like watching down parachute away.

And now he sits in a lounge chair, here, but not here,
Grasping at the vanishing point of a memory,
Trapped by his dis-ease and the blank beige walls.

And now we walk the aisle together, she and I, arm in arm,
Held together by our life-not-as-planned,
A life of encrusted fingernails and distant eyes
And forgotten words. And forgotten. Everything.

And I want to remember how singular this moment is,
At the altar, surrounded by all who love her,
A congregation of family and friends and saints.
Because I know he is here too, spectacled large grey eyes,
Standing tall on his runner's legs, here in our hearts,
Here in his flash-forward memory. Here.
Watching this dandelion-strong daughter of ours,
In down-like tulle, parachute away.

❧

From the beginning, I strove to have Harvey remain an integral part of our lives and include him in our daily activities as well as larger events. The temptation to just do it all by myself was there, of course; it would be easier and take less time. But where was the humanity in that for Harvey? Plus, I needed his help as much as he needed to give it. So, as I've said, we transitioned the cooking, the laundry, and the finances all gradually, with me leaning on him at the first, but with him leaning on me more and more as time progressed. I purposely planned vacations that I thought we could enjoy as a family, choosing to include Harvey in this part of our lives as well. He also attended funerals and weddings, with me by his side to help translate and communicate.

Having Harvey at Elena and Brett's wedding was difficult to orchestrate. At that point in Harvey's illness, he wasn't aware of what was happening, but we knew that he would have wanted to be there for her. And we did it for Elena's sake, and for mine and Christina's. And it was worth it!

Your loved one needs to feel included and needed. In daily chores, consider asking him to help you with a small task, maybe folding the laundry or stirring the soup, something that he can actually accomplish. This gives him a sense of purpose and of contributing to the household. Asking him for his help lets him know that you need him. His skills may not be perfect, but that is not the goal. Also consider saying, "Let's do it together" as you work side by side, even when he is no longer able to help.

❧

PRACTICE

1. What small tasks can you ask your loved one to do? Consider how you can ask for his help in a way that makes him feel useful and worthy. Do you get frustrated with his lack of skill? If so, back away and reassess what you and he really need from this interaction. Create a song playlist to enjoy while you are together.

2. If you have a big event in the future, such as a wedding or a family reunion, plan ahead as far as you can to make the event as enjoyable as possible for everyone. You may decide that your loved one cannot attend, and that is OK. Have contingency plans if things don't go according to the plan.

3. Play together. Recalling your loved one's favorite activities as a child, create moments where you can enjoy just being together—playing catch, dancing, coloring, building with blocks. You may have to adapt the activities to her current abilities.

Pneumonia is the End-Stage Dementia Patient's Friend

Once Harvey had the added sitters with him during daylight hours at the third nursing home, he was no longer getting in trouble, and care was seamless. Of course, he continued to decline, inch by inch. He began having seizures, despite being on medication, each one lasting longer than the last, and taking an even longer time to recover from them. His walking became slower, his posture now permanently hunched over, especially at his neck, and he would, for days at a time, lean severely to the right in his chair, and more alarmingly, while walking. He brightened with less enthusiasm to my visits, but continued to respond to his name, though he could no longer speak it. He could no longer clap along with our song. He slept more and more during the day. I got phone calls occasionally from the nursing home that he had fallen during the night, the staff finding him on the floor. When I asked for guardrails on his bed, they initially refused, saying it would create a hazard if his head lodged between the bed and the rails. Eventually, they relented and acquired a hospital bed with rails for him and a padded mat beside the bed.

But it wasn't all depressing during this period. Because Harvey had sitters to engage him all the time, he became more alert and interactive when he wasn't sleeping. They walked the halls together and listened to music. I had purchased a small boom box and brought his favorite CDs, mostly 1970s light rock—James Taylor, Fleetwood Mac, and Steely Dan. His beloved Bruce Springsteen was too jarring, and he became agitated when I tried to play "Born to Run." The sitters and certified nursing assistants (CNAs) at the nursing home noted that playing soothing music seemed to calm him when he needed his clothes changed, and it helped put him to sleep at night.

Harvey's fifty-eighth birthday fell in this time frame. The girls, their guys, and I contrived a party of sorts, more for us, I suspect, than for Harvey. That Friday evening, Elena and Brett arrived with a pizza, Christina and Phil brought balloons and a cake, and I showed up with a cooler of beer. We snuck the beer onto the outdoor patio of his dementia unit and gathered around a wrought iron table. (Don't worry, I only poured Harvey a half cup of beer, and he drank it right up!) He was cute and funny this evening, interacting with us occasionally, laughing appropriately even. At one point Christina praised him for being such a good father, and with sincere humility, he bowed his head and said, "Thank you." Amazing! We loved this so much that Christina repeated the compliment two more times.

Lois passed away about this same time, but we never told Harvey, and of course, he never asked about her. Actually, Christina reported that when she and Dennis were visiting him during Lois's last week, Dennis did try to tell Harvey that their mother was "passing," but it made no impact on him, and made Christina feel terribly uncomfortable. My dreams of the two of them interacting once he had moved to this nursing home never materialized, though we did get them together occasionally. However, it distressed Lois too badly and we stopped. She would say things like, "What's wrong with him?" or "Who is that? That's not Harvey."

Lois contracted pneumonia, was hospitalized, and then seemed to recover. When she started deteriorating again, Dennis decided to keep her in the nursing home for treatment. She didn't respond to the antibiotics and declined to the point that hospice was called. Our daughters and I got to say goodbye, and I sang some hymns to her. She died peacefully in her bed, with her daughter-in-law Jane holding her hand. Elena planned to visit that morning, and actually came into the room soon after Lois had passed away. After the small, sweet funeral and graveside service, the girls and I ate dinner together and reminisced about their beloved grandmother.

Almost exactly eight years after Harvey's official diagnosis, he was no longer able to walk. This former marathon runner still had strong leg muscles, according to reports from physical therapy, but his brain no longer communicated what it wanted his legs to do. It took two CNAs to lift him off a chair, then carry/guide his upright body to and from the dining room. At any moment of this three-person shamble, Harvey might suddenly bend forward as if to sit down, causing the CNAs to have to yank him up by the back waistband of his pants. Because he was no longer ambulatory, he was given a wheelchair and was moved to a skilled nursing floor, actually the same floor on which his parents had resided, and where we were familiar with the staff. This unit had floor-to-ceiling windows in the dining room, and the staff would wheel Harvey into this bright space every day. And because he was no longer wandering or having behavioral issues, he no longer needed the extra sitters.

About two months after the move to the new skilled nursing unit, Harvey declined further, sleeping most of the day, rousing only for mealtimes—meals were completely fed to him now. He began to forget to swallow, water dribbling out of his mouth, and we would have to gently stroke his throat to coax a swallow reflex. I thought now might be a good time to bring in hospice, but the unit nurse said that since he was still eating well it wasn't time. Maybe I should have pushed for it, but I chose not to; he was being cared for compassionately and appropriately by the staff.

On a busy Monday at my office, I answered a phone call from Harvey's nurse practitioner. She said that it appeared to the staff and to her that Harvey had had an unwitnessed seizure over the weekend, because there had been a big decline in his alertness, with him not even rousing for meals. On Wednesday morning, she called again: he had developed a fever, some shortness of breath, and congestion in his chest. The nurse practitioner thought that he had probably aspirated retained food particles during the seizure, inhaling food into his lungs that he had not swallowed, and that he now had pneumonia, technically aspiration pneumonia. After giving me her assessment, she asked, "I know that your husband is a DNR (do not resuscitate), but do you want us to treat his pneumonia, or do you want comfort measures only now?"

Wow! We're doing this now? On a regular Wednesday morning? Ideas and options flashed through my mind. They could treat him for pneumonia in the nursing home, and he might recover. But to what end? Back to what baseline? What good was that? Who would that serve? Harvey and I had living wills, and his clearly stated that he did not want treatment if he had a terminal illness. I took a deep breath and said, "Comfort measures only."

The nursing home called in hospice, and I phoned the girls, my parents and sisters, Nancy, Dennis, and a few close friends. I was still in charge and in control of it all, managing phone calls and texts from family and friends, taking care of my patients' needs at the office, making sure our daughters were emotionally grounded. I didn't have time to fall apart. It almost seemed as if I were observing what was happening as a spectator. I'm told I made good, clear decisions during this process, but I don't remember the details. "You're so strong, Renée!" I've heard that sentiment a thousand times. But what else could I be?

Since Wednesdays were my half days, I was able to leave the office at noon and go straight to the nursing home. I found Harvey somewhat alert and moving in vague, nonpurposeful movements. Christina and Elena joined me fairly quickly, both of them leaving their jobs early to be with their father and me. I explained all that I knew about the situation. The hospice nurse arrived, as did the chaplain of the nursing home. The hospice nurse explained that the usual course of aspiration pneumonia was three to five days. She said that they were going to use morphine to curb his pain from the dying process and loraze-pam to calm him. He also had oxygen and was placed on an air mattress. When we left that evening, Harvey was comfortably sleeping.

I had to work the next day, Thursday, but I left at noon and went straight to the nursing home. When I walked into Harvey's room, I found him lying flat on his back, mouth wide open and not breathing. "Breathe, Harv!" I whispered. He took a deep shuddering breath, and started breathing again. Then his breathing slowed, and again he stopped breathing for what seemed a lifetime. From a clinical perspective, I knew this was apneic breathing, but on a personal level, it was terrifying. I rallied my clinician's brain and timed his breaths and apneic spells. They were consistent across the several cycles that I timed. Putting on my doctor hat gave me some distance at this moment, alone with my husband who was now actively dying. I could objectively view what was happening and not be over-come with grief. There was more disbelief than grief. We're really doing this now? As if I hadn't been expecting it.

Elena and Christina came soon after, and Nancy arrived with a tub of body butter and led us in a ritual of re-membering Harvey. Because his memory was broken, thus dis-membered, we re-membered for him, pulling his memories back together and presenting them to him in turn. As we rubbed the silky lotion into his skin, each of us spoke to Harvey, sharing our memories of him, and massaging him in gentle circular motions.

Friday morning, I arrived to find Harvey breathing regularly, if shallowly. The girls, Brett, and Phil came soon after, then Dennis, and later Nancy. We sat by the bedside and were gentle with each other. The girls asked Dennis to describe Harvey as a child, and he told us tales of bicycles and dogs and swimming and scouting. Dennis was re-membering for Harvey too. Friends came and went, some bringing our meals to us. Through the day, Harvey's breathing patterns would vary, with light, shallow breaths and spells of the same apneic pattern. We started to see some pale purplish discoloration on his knees and elbows, but his coloring was good otherwise. The medications made him completely flaccid, the only thing moving was his chest. I sang hymns to him late into the evening, and we gave him permission to leave. That night, as we were preparing to go home for the night, Christina couldn't give herself permission to leave his bedside. She worried that her father might pass away, alone, while we were gone, and she wasn't sure if she could come back to see his body if that happened overnight. So she and Phil gathered lounge chairs and wheelchairs and attempted to sleep through the night.

We all returned the next day to hold vigil. After all the visitors said goodbye that evening, we who were left—Elena, Christina, Brett, Phil, and I—began to mentally prepare to return to our homes. It was harder to leave Harvey and each other that night. We needed to be there together—talking, or not, singing, praying, being present.

Catching my eye, Brett conveyed that I should look at Harvey. He was breathing very shallowly now, in short, quick inhalations, but very few exhalations, a type of breathing pattern that the hospice nurse termed "fish out of water."

I gathered the girls onto his bed and told them that I thought this was the end. I grabbed one of Harvey's hands, and Christina the other. I sang, "Surely the presence of the Lord is in this place. I can feel His mighty power and His grace. I can hear the brush of angel wings; I see glory on each face. Surely the presence of the Lord is in this place." Then I prayed, thanking God for the gift of Harvey in our lives and in this world. I commended him back to the Source of All. Then, while Elena and I sang two verses of "Amazing Grace," Harvey breathed his last breath, and incredibly, Christina felt her father squeeze her hand. It was his last gift to her. And what an incredible gift it was to all four of us to be together in this most holy of moments, singing him home across still waters. I treasure now the poignancy that we were together at the births of these amazing daughters, and then again, at the end of Harvey's singular, precious life.

☙

I hadn't the time or mental energy to prepare for what would happen after Harvey passed away. I knew only that he was to be cremated. The girls and I decided that since there wasn't a body to bury, we could plan a service in a time frame that suited as many people as possible. We chose to have it three weeks later, in the beautiful old sanctuary of our church, in downtown Birmingham. It would be on a Saturday, so that more people would be able to attend. Elena wrote the obituary, and it included the plans for the service as well as requests that donations be made to our local chapter of the Alzheimer's Foundation. The girls and I met with Nancy to plan the service, and I asked her to officiate in her capacity as a United Methodist clergyperson. We decided on hymns and scripture and who we wanted to include. Because we knew there would be a lot of guests, I wanted to feed them well and have a chance to visit with as many as possible. My parents offered to plan the reception, and I gladly accepted. Christina began creating a slideshow of photos of her father to project during the reception, and I gathered Harvey's diploma, stethoscope, favorite books and CDs, a marathon medal, and framed photos for a remembrance table.

The service was perfect and everything that we had hoped it would be. I had asked a friend, an accomplished pianist who had played for Harvey's and my wedding, to play for the service. She led with Cat Stevens's version of "Morning Has Broken," another of Harvey's favorites. Our pastor opened the service with beautiful words, addressing the 350 people present. Then Elena read a lovely prayer that she had written, and our friend Bill, the friend who had shepherded Harvey while I had band practice, read a selection of scripture. Our previous pastor spoke, then Nancy delivered her eulogy, speaking of Harvey's healing presence in all our lives. Next was a succession of witnesses from different aspects of Harvey's life. His friend Chris spoke of Harvey as a friend, an older gentleman spoke of him as a physician, Christina spoke of him as a father, and I spoke of him as a husband.

I told the gathered congregation, for it was a holy time and space, about how Harvey and I met, fell in love, and then created our perfectly balanced life together as equal partners. I spoke briefly about his Alzheimer's disease and his inability to talk about it.

Earlier, while preparing my eulogy, I finally forgave him for not discussing the diagnosis with me for all those years. I had come to realize that while he was at home all those days alone, he was surely processing the implications of the disease, and he neither wanted nor needed to talk to me about it. Maybe he was even shielding me from his pain.

I told the story of the last minutes of his life, how the four of us were all together, singing "Amazing Grace" and holding hands. I closed by sharing my realization of the wonderful bookended moment of my grabbing his hand and holding on tight at the end, just as he had done at our beginning, on our first date.

ᴄ⁄ᴐ

Alzheimer's disease is a terminal illness. A patient *can* die from it, but usually, a complication of dementia is the ultimate cause of death, as Harvey's pneumonia was. A fall can be fatal, especially if a head injury is involved. Most elderly patients with Alzheimer's disease have other age-related illnesses and may die of those complications.

When the end comes, I can almost guarantee that you won't be ready. And when it comes, you will respond as differently as you are different in the world. Own that. Your grief will be your own. You can't plan it. You might anticipate it, but in the end, you will experience it how you experience it. It will be what it will be.

I do recommend having a living will. You can draw up a simple one online, or you may prefer to ask a lawyer to draft one for you. The standard ones include only issues around feeding, fluids, and resuscitation. The best-case scenario would be to have a discussion with your loved one before the diagnosis of dementia is even made, listing his wishes in a document, stating clearly what medical modalities would be allowed should he develop a terminal illness. Once a diagnosis of dementia is made, it would be best to have another thorough discussion about end-of-life issues. Make sure all family members are aware of the loved one's wishes so that there are no surprises at the end.

ಎ

PRACTICE

1. Visualize what the "perfect death" may look like for your family member. Who would be present? What music or sounds would there be? Consider a meaningful bedside ritual that will help you and your family members say goodbye.

2. Start thinking about your loved one's funeral or memorial service. It may sound morbid to you now, but the more you plan ahead, the easier it will be. Think about who you would want to speak. What music or scripture, if either, would you and your loved one like? Maybe you can even plan this together early in the disease process.

3. Plan how you will communicate important transitions with friends and relatives. How much are you willing to share regarding an acute illness, hospice care, death? Who in your village can you rely on to spread information? What parameters might you need regarding visits?

Epilogue

You Are So Strong

I went back to work too soon. I even stupidly went to church the Sunday after Harvey died, November 1, All Saints' Day. Sheesh! I couldn't see what else I needed to do with more time off. I had gotten everything squared away with the cremation, the planning of the service, and some initial financial paperwork. I suspect I just wanted to keep busy and not stop to process all that had happened, but I couched it in terms of "I'm fine! I've been expecting this for some time." And I thought that my patients needed me back in the office.

What I didn't realize was that my patients needed me back in the office in a way I wasn't expecting. They needed to grieve. I had compiled a list of patients that I knew would want to be told when Harvey died, and my staff called them once he had passed away, but we invariably missed some. Every day for weeks, I hugged my patients, and listened as they talked through tears about how much Harvey had meant to them.

What really threw me were the patients who greeted me with a smile and said, "So, how's Dr. Harvey?" I had to tell these unsuspecting souls that he had passed away, taking them completely by surprise. And so we grieved together, my patients and I, healing each other in the process. My staff posted his obituary at the check-in desk and had copies available, and many patients came to the memorial service.

I was inundated with cards, flowers, and small gifts. I don't know the final total, but a sizable amount of money was donated to Alzheimer's of Central Alabama in Harvey's memory. We had meals brought to us for a solid week, and it was a gift to be able to share these meals together with the girls and their guys. My Sunday school class offered to bring meals, and I don't remember saying this, but evidently I asked that they be spaced out once a week. Well, what a blessing that was. Weekly family meals together continued through December. We loved the regularity of that so much that we have continued to schedule a meal together every other week, taking turns with the cooking, just as Harvey and I had done before his diagnosis.

The overarching comment I have gotten over the entire eight years has been, "Renée, you are so strong!" Seemed like a good title for this book even. I guess I am, but what other option was there? I wasn't going to run away. I didn't cry in public often, so most people didn't really know how devastating it all was to me. And I had to be strong for our daughters. They were so young. And for Harvey. I couldn't very well dissolve into tears when his fate was so much worse than mine. So I wrote. I filled six journals with my laments and fears, and chronicled Harvey's symptoms. And along the way, I learned to surf, riding the waves that kept coming, threatening to overturn me. And I had a lot of people in my village, rooting for me and helping me. I stayed upright through it all.

I *am* strong. I know that I am. I am strong because I have deep roots, embedded in the rich soil of my faith, my family, and my community. I am strong because my trunk is strong, yet flexible enough to bend in the wind. My trunk represents myself, the core of who I am; it's how I was born and how I was raised to be. I am strong because my branches reach far, providing shelter for my daughters, my patients, and Harvey when he was alive. I am strong because my leaves reach for the sun, the Source, absorbing energy when I remember to spend time in God's presence. But I am not a lone tree. I am in a forest of trees, some bigger and stronger than myself, giving me shelter under their branches. I am made even stronger because my roots intertwine with the roots of all the other trees in my forest community. We hold each other up, braced and secure. This forest is stronger than the individual trees. Not even the tsunami of Alzheimer's disease could knock this forest down.

Acknowledgments

So many people to thank! I am so full of gratitude for all the wonderful folks who walked alongside Harvey, Elena, Christina, and me through the entirety of this unplanned journey into Alzheimer's world.

To my family of origin: Thank you for your ears that heard all my concerns and for loving me even when I was nothing but shattered. To my parents, who "Harvey-sat" so that I could attend a dementia support group. To my sister, who opened up her home whenever we needed a place to escape and who accompanied me on the search for memory care units.

To our daughters, Elena and Christina: I truly don't know how you grew up to be such amazing women given the adolescence you had. I know this experience shaped you, and it seems to have shaped you for the good. When I try to imagine what your lives would be like without this experience, I can't conceive of anything better than what you are right now. I am so proud that you both have made careers of helping the vulnerable. Thank you, too, to Brett and Phil for embracing our family and loving these daughters so well.

To Dennis: I'm still not sure how you managed your own and your parents' health issues as well as all of their financial issues during the eight years that Harvey and I were unable to assist you. Well done! Thank you, too, for your faithful visits with Harvey (and your gift of a chocolate milkshake for him every time!).

To our friends: Nancy, Hanna, and Amy, you dissident daughters were the first to hear my fears, and you never let go of me. Bill, you will never know how much it saved me to be able to continue to play the keyboard in the Loft while you shepherded Harvey. Chris, your long-distance relationship with Harvey and me was a gift I hadn't expected, but treasure deeply.

To our First Church family: The pastors, staff, and congregation were always there to love our family through Harvey's illness. I cannot imagine a church more willing to accept and love anyone that walks through her doors. Even if they are wearing pajamas.

To our caregivers: Caroline and SchRonda, you slipped into our family with such ease! I am so grateful for the two years that you gave me the peace of mind to leave Harvey in your hands. The staff at the memory care units, geriatric psychiatry units, the home health nurses, and the hospice nurses all deserve way more than they are currently afforded. This needs to change!

To Pam and all the staff and volunteers at CARES: You guys are the best! You opened up your arms and your hearts to love Harvey exactly as he was. If you ever get another participant half as competitive at balloon volleyball as Harvey was, let me know.

To the staff of Double Oak Family Medicine: We were a family, weren't we?! It was a privilege to work alongside you. You grieved almost as much as I did when Harvey had to retire, and you supported me in innumerable ways as I tried to balance my life as physician, mother, and caregiver. I am so proud of the work we did, and how well we ministered to our patients.

To our patients at Double Oak Family Medicine: Wow! What an honor it was to have each of you place your trust in Harvey and me! I was especially moved by all you patients of Harvey's who gave me a chance to prove that I might be as good a physician as he was. Those were big shoes to fill. I am so grateful for all your honest concern for Harvey and me. It was a blessing to hear how much he meant to you and to be reminded almost daily of the care he had for you.

To those who helped to bring this book into the world: First, to Dehryl—without your vision board session, I really don't think this book would exist. When I actually said the words, "I think I want to write a book," you took it seriously, even if I meant it only as a pie-in-the-sky dream. Together with Sonja, you guys kept me accountable and on track. Hanna, thank you for your help and ideas for the practice sections. Kelly Notaras, your book, *The Book You Were Born to Write*, and the Kripalu Authors Group were such rich sources of information. Even as I inwardly groaned at the mention of "platform building," I came to understand that everything you taught was accurate and true. My editor, Ben LeRoy, was the first person to read my manuscript without first knowing our story. His feedback gave me the courage to know that this book was worth the effort. Blake, my author website shines because of your talent.

To all the caregivers, advocates, and persons living with Alzheimer's disease and other dementias: You are seen, you are heard, and you are loved. May we one day soon see the scientific breakthroughs for which we have all been longing.

About the Author

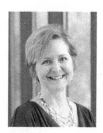

Renée Brown Harmon, MD, resides in Birmingham, Alabama, where she has recently retired from a twenty-nine-year career in family medicine. She and her husband shared responsibilities at their medical practice, and at their home with two daughters, until Alzheimer's disease forced his retirement.